The Jo[y of]

Bedwetting

... a different view on bedwetting ...

© 2017

Forrest Grant

Title: The Joy of Bedwetting

Author: Forrest Grant

Editor: Michael Bent

Publisher: AB Discovery

© 2017

www.abdiscovery.com.au

Other Books from Forrest Grant

The Joy of Bedwetting
Overlapping Stains
The Babies and Bedwetters of Baker St
The Bedwetter's Travel Guide
The Joy of Nappies
Growing up a Bedwetter
Three Sissy Babies

Other Books from AB Discovery

Six Misfits
Six Misfits – A man and his dog
The Six Misfits – the seventh misfit
The Adult Baby Identity – coming out as ABDL
The Adult Baby Identity – Healing Childhood Wounds
Living with Chrissie – my life as an Adult Baby
The Adult Baby Identity – a self-help guide
The Adult Baby Identity – the dissociation spectrum
Becoming Me – The Journey of Self-acceptance
Living happily as an Adult Baby
Adult Babies and Diaper Lovers – a guidebook
There's still a baby in my bed!
So, Your teenager is wearing diapers!
Where Big Babies Live

Home Detention
Adult Babies: Psychology and Practices
Coffee with Rosie
Being an Adult Baby
The Three Chambers
A Brother for Samantha
Mummy's Diary
The Hypnotist
Chosen
The Snoop
The Washing Line
My Baby Callum
A Baby for Felicity
The Regression of Baby Noah
A Baby for Melissa and her Mother
Baby Solutions
Discharged into Infancy
The English Baby
A Mother's Love
The Psychiatrist and her Patient
The Reluctant Baby
The Book Club Baby
The Rehab Regression
The Daycare Regression
A Woman's Guide to Babying Her Partner
The ABC of Baby Women
Me, Myself, Christine
Diaper Discipline and Dominance
The Epitome of Love
Australian Baby: a life of nappies, bottles and struggles
Fear and Joy: a life in and out of nappies
The Fulltime, Permanent Adult Infant

Contents

Introduction

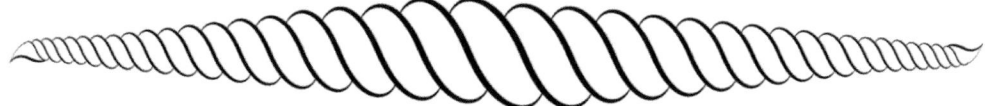

I WET THE BED. I am not ashamed of it.

I WET THE BED EVERY NIGHT. I don't feel the overwhelming need to change this.

I WET MY SHEETS, PILLOW AND MATTRESS. I find it both natural and comforting.

I WET THE BED in my sleep, and it feels both right and normal.

I WET THE BED no matter where I sleep because I am a bedwetter

I WET THE BED and I am proud of it

I WET THE BED and it is an achievement, not a failure

I WET THE BED and it is not just for children. It is for me as well

I WET THE BED and it is who I am

Bedwetting is one of those things that few talk about, few admit to and yet is incredibly common. It is easy to believe the fiction that only young children – and pre-schoolers at that – wet the bed. The truth, however, is that bedwetting is remarkably common, especially given what it is.

However, bedwetting is not necessarily a disaster for some people. It may, in fact, be something they are ambivalent about or even seek pleasure in! It is easy to subscribe to the societal belief that bedwetting is 'wrong'.

The truth of more accurate and more modern statistics is that a *lot* of people wet the bed and a surprising number never really stop their nightly wettings. Certainly, the large majority of children and teens grow out of it, but still there remains a very large number who wet their sheets or night diapers anything from once a week to seven times a week. It is not what we often want to believe. For some reason, bedwetting is something people do not share about with anyone, even preferring to discuss deep intimate secrets and problems long before admitting to wetting their bed. Historical instances record where bedwetting was grossly under-reported by parents and was only revealed by doctor's interviews. Deeply personal or traumatic events are often reported before bedwetting is. It is viewed by so many as a personal failure or the failure as a parent. And yet the simple fact is that heaps and heaps of people wet the bed. And not just children. A surprising number of adults wet the bed, and many are deeply ashamed of it. This book, of course, takes the other angle in that if you wet the bed, you should be proud of it! It is not a failure of any kind. If you don't want to wet the bed, there are super-effective diapers available to look after that for you. If bedwetting is a good thing in your mind, then you are not alone.

If you want some data, there is an Appendix at the end of this book with a detailed set of data about bedwetting and you will be blown away by how common it is and yet, it is still something most people refuse to talk about.

In this book, I want to discuss bedwetting in a positive, life-affirming way. There is no shame in bedwetting. The shame comes from other people and you have no need to be embarrassed or ashamed of the wet sheets or wet diapers that you wake up to every morning. Let them in fact, be your badge of honour.

Perhaps you are one that rather than wanting to stop bedwetting, you want to *start* it. This book is for you as well. Why should bedwetting be something you can't stop? Why can't it be a lifestyle choice, a preference or a goal? Why can't it be something we actively choose to do and start? In this book, we will explore bedwetting in a positive way. My own personal experience is that of a near life-time bedwetter and I am not at all ashamed of it nor do I think anyone else should be. I will discuss my philosophy of bedwetting as we go on.

Diapers or Wet Sheets?

Probably the most obvious question or issue about bedwetting is the issue of diapers (or nappies). Essentially it is the question of using protection or not.

Typically, a bedwetter will be kept in diapers for some time while growing up, but then have them taken away, even though bedwetting is still occurring. In previous generations, the absence of diapers for older children made the question a moot point, but now, with a vast array of diapers for older children, the question is one that parents still have options with. A lot of parents take diapers away, hoping that the discomfort of wet sheets will motivate their child to stop bedwetting. Typically, it is just a vain hope that is rarely rewarded. Children and teens normally just stop bedwetting when they are ready - either physically or emotionally. The wet sheet discomfort usually doesn't make much difference. When you've known nothing different, a wet sheet is not that motivating, especially in warm climates. It might even perversely be a place of comfort and security and not unlike a security blanket.

So, as adult bedwetters, what do we want? Wet diapers or wet sheets? It is very much a personal choice and for many, they choose both at times. So, what are the advantages and disadvantages?

Advantages

Diapers: they are clearly very convenient and especially so if you use disposables. Your bedwetting is dispensed within a few moments as the wet diaper is removed, bagged and binned. If you wear cloth, it just goes into the diaper pail ready for washing later on. Easy as.

Wet sheets: Incredibly easy to manage if you are happy to just let the sheet dry out during the day and wash weekly (or less) as normal. No extra cost or effort involved. If you enjoy a stained sheet and the implicit statement of pride, wet sheets are truly remarkable. They are ironically, the easiest choice, if workload is the issue.

Disadvantages

Diapers: they are expensive and can be bulky. They take away evidence of bedwetting for others (or yourself) to see. If bedwetting is something you are proud of, a disposable diaper will take away all evidence of your bedwetting far too quickly.

Wet sheets: unless you are comfortable in a wet bed, you may find wet sheets a negative experience for sleep. What some do not understand is that after years in wet sheets, comfort is not that hard to find. For some, a dry bed feels odd!

In normal life, bedwetters may choose a combination of both. Warm weather may make wetting the sheets a good and easy option while in cooler weather, diapers may be the better choice.

What should I choose?

The important thing is to *have* a choice. Allow yourself to choose diapered or un-diapered bedwetting. Experiment over time with each option and see what you like best and when it suits you.

Wet sheets are nothing to be embarrassed by. You are in good company and a fairly large company at that. Likewise, a bag of wet diapers is nothing to feel shame over. A huge number of people just like you are wearing them to bed and waking saturated but contented.

I will say, however, that for many people, until you have had some large wet puddles on your sheets, your bedwetting is still a bit artificial. That might be a bit harsh, but there is nothing to compare with the visual effect of soaking wet and highly visible wet patches on your sheets. After all 'bedwetting' does mean wetting your bed, not just your diaper.

The Question of the Mattress – part one

Most of us grew up with a waterproof sheet covering our mattress. In recent years, however, these are being made from discreet and noiseless materials meaning that the friend sitting on your bed would never know you wet the bed. When I was growing up, however, the rather ignorant powers-that-be never even made waterproofs for beds past toddler size and so generations grew up with rubber and then plastic sheets over the mattress that were too small and often ineffective. And plastic sheets after a few years of torrential bedwetting became brittle and crackly, thus loudly announcing to all that your bed was a bedwetter's bed. To add to the experience, these waterproofs were not fitted, but mere sheets that could move thus allowing the mattress to still get wet quite often. A pee-stained mattress was therefore inevitable and for many children growing up, a part of life.

So, should we as bedwetters still use waterproof protection over our mattress?

Common sense might say yes, but why should common-sense matter?

If you have the ability to dry your mattress out at least weekly, should you be forced to cover it? If you enjoy wet sheets and are proud of it, why should you prevent your mattress from getting the pee-stains as well?

Simply, the choice is yours to make.

Even if you wear diapers to bed, they will from time to time leak, sometimes extensively. Your unprotected mattress will get wet and be a witness to your night-time wetting. If you don't wear diapers to bed, your unprotected mattress will get very wet every night. It will get very stained and be an unchanging statement that you are a bedwetter!

What you choose to do is up to you. You may choose a combination of these options. In a hot dry climate or season where drying out sheets and mattresses is not very difficult, you could eschew all protection entirely and let your sheets, mattress and pillow get as wet as you like. In cooler climates or seasons, you may want some level of protection, either all the time or occasionally.

The main point is that protecting the mattress is not an essential element of good and responsible bedwetting. What you choose to do is up to you and there is no right answer other than for your bladder to empty while you are in bed. The level of protection you provide is an individual choice.

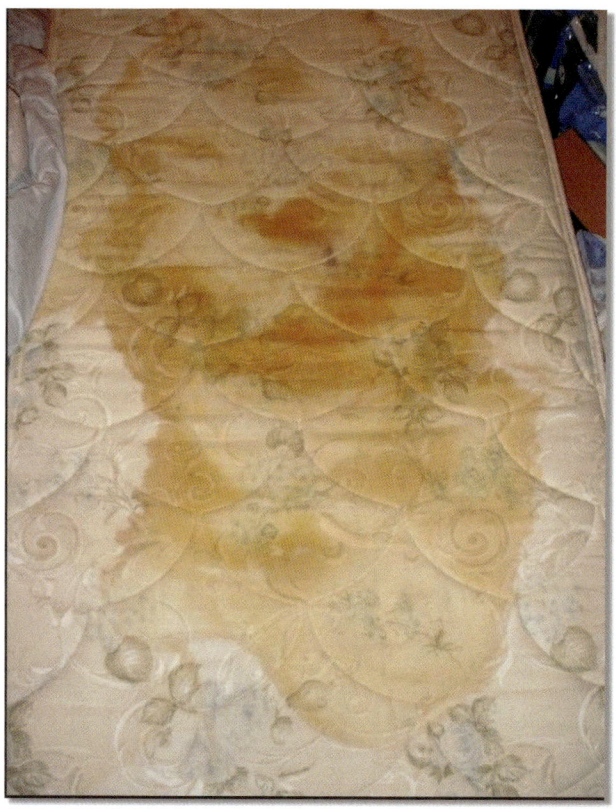

What really is bedwetting?

This might sound like a bizarre question to begin with, but it isn't really. The clinical term is enuresis, but we normally just call it bedwetting.

If I wear diapers to bed, is it still bedwetting? Yes, it is. You are in bed and you are wetting, therefore it is bedwetting.

If I deliberately wet when I am in bed, is it still bedwetting? Yes, it is! Once again, you are in bed and you are wetting and therefore it is still bedwetting. If I only wet once a month, is it still bedwetting? Yes, it is. The act of peeing in your bed, even occasionally, means you can consider yourself to be a bedwetter.

The activity of bedwetting can carry a very large emotional overtone that can confuse and discourage people. This is what we need to let go of in this book.

If you wet while you are in bed, either in a diaper or on the sheets, you are a real bedwetter!

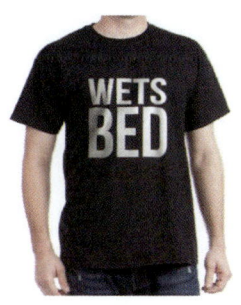

That is the basic truth. If you pee while you are in bed, then you are a bedwetter. You don't have to be asleep to be a bedwetter. You don't need to wear the literal teeshirt to be a bedwetter, although if you want to, go right ahead!

Having said that, there are a lot of people who really, really want to experience bedwetting while asleep. I understand that, because despite what I've said above, for many people, having to deliberately wet their bed diminishes the experience somewhat. They know that they are a bedwetter already, but what they want is what they call *'genuine bedwetting'*. The first thing to do is to accept that even if you are awake when wetting your bed, it is still 'genuine bedwetting'. What you want is the *premium experience* of waking up in the morning refreshed and... soaking wet without any effort to be so and no memory of wetting.

In our next chapter, we are going to look at ways to achieve *premium bedwetting*.

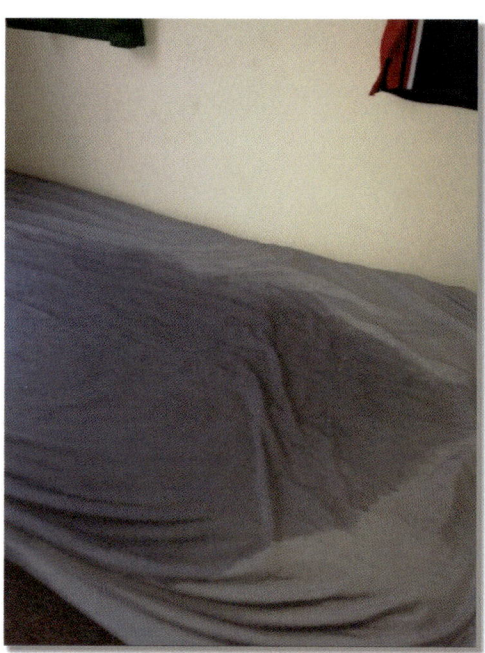

Learning to wet the bed

Well, here we are, wanting to learn to wet the bed. The first thing we need to discuss is our goals.

For most of us, the desire we share is that we can wet the bed at this level – completely accidentally, during sleep with no effort, regardless of circumstances or how much we have been drinking. We want to wet our beds effortlessly like we did as toddlers. This is what we call *premium bedwetting*. It is the very best outcome, but it is also the most difficult to achieve and certainly difficult in the short term. Perhaps it could be called *toddler bedwetting!*

The next level down is easy bedwetting. This level is where we wet the bed semi-deliberately. By that, I mean that when a full bladder wakes us during the night, we quickly and easily just relax and let the pee flow out naturally and easily, but while we are awake. This is a good stage to be in because when it is easy to do, it becomes second nature and you don't even need to wake up very much. It is also a step towards premium bedwetting.

The next level down is *deliberate bedwetting.* This level is different from 'easy' bedwetting in that the wetting is not easy and natural, but rather requires effort and concentration and an intellectual decision to wet your bed. While this is not the best solution for many, it is where many who seek to return to bedwetting, start. To be honest, it is not a bad place to be where you wet your bed every night by conscious choice and effort. It is a solid achievement to do this and one to be proud of because 'wannabes' will baulk at the first squirt and the first wet patch. Real bedwetters – like you aim to be – will find the outcome of deliberate bedwetting to be enjoyable and a source of pride. It is also a great place to build upon. Every long march needs a first step. This is the first step.

This chapter brings up some ideas and suggestions and a skeleton program to achieve the goal of wetting during the night.

Sheets or Diapers?

The first issue to address is 'sheets or diapers'? Do you want to wet your sheets or your diapers? In reality, it is usually both, but you will absolutely need to get ready for soaked bedsheets at times. You cannot really develop as a bedwetter if you are not ready and prepared for some wet sheets – either from diaper leakage or from unprotected wetting. Wet bedding is the occasional outcome of even the best-protected bedwetter.

Becoming a premium bedwetter again is not a simple process. Sadly, toilet training is something that becomes deeply ingrained in us and is extremely difficult to alter. So, if you want to be a premium bedwetter again then you will need to do the work.

So, which do you want? Wet sheets...

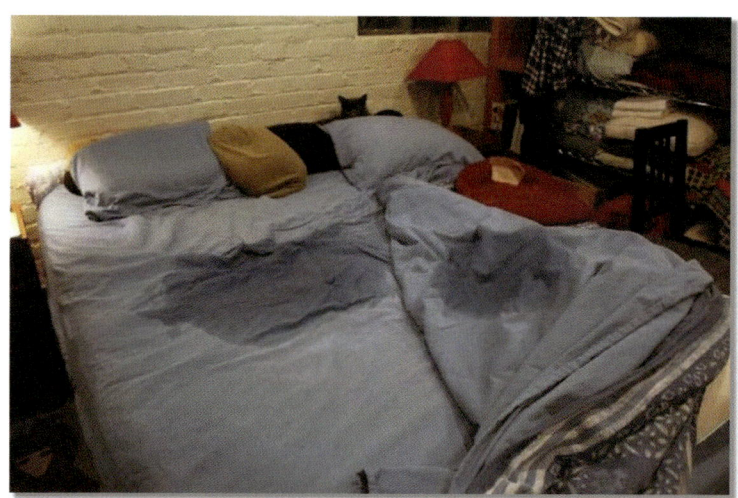

Or wet diapers?

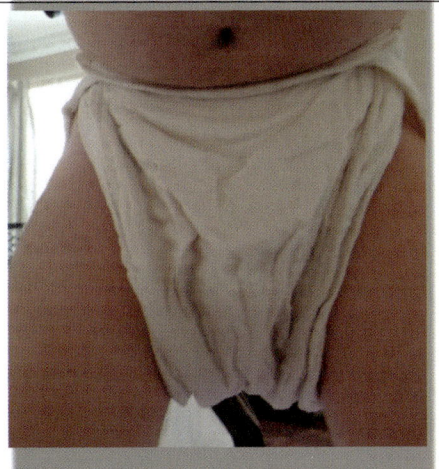

To be honest, you don't get to be totally protected at night even in diapers. Anyone who has actually worn diapers to bed knows that there are still accidents. Sometimes you leak outside a nappy because you tossed and turned overnight and the protection is not complete. Other times you simply wet so much that it is never going to all stay inside the diaper. And with disposables, in particular, sleeping on your side gives you less protection than on your back or front. And sometimes the nappy comes off during the night. And so, you end up with this – a wet bed <u>and</u> a wet nappy.

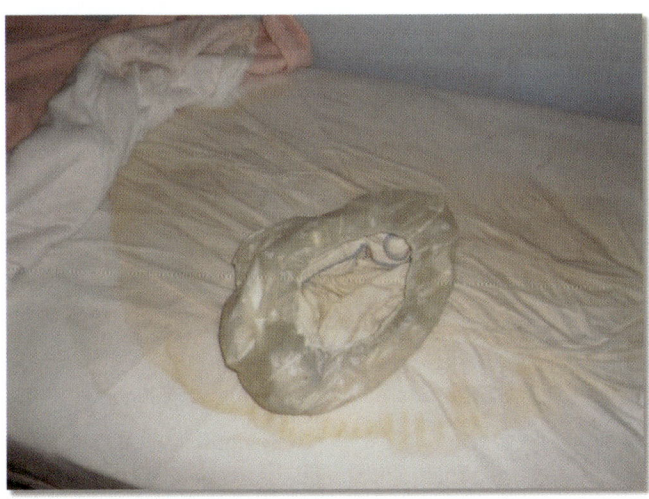

Setting goals

The first thing to do is to set goals and this is incredibly important. I know that for most people the goal will be 'to wet while I sleep every night'. That is a worthy goal, but also the top-end and one that is difficult to achieve. I need to be honest here and remind you that premium toddler-style bedwetting can be a difficult thing to achieve, albeit very worthwhile and desirable.

Remember, if you achieve the goal of premium bedwetting then you will wet when you sleep – including naps or falling asleep in front of the TV at night. So be wary of what you are looking for and make sure you are willing to accept the responsibilities that go along with your goal. Even if you don't wear diapers during the night, you will need to have some diapers around for when you travel or on trips where you will fall asleep in another's bed or in a plane or wherever.

Setting the scene

The first thing you should do is to set the scene properly for your bedwetting. If you want to begin with diapered bedwetting, then get your night absorbency diapers and put them out in your bedroom... in the open. Put the packets of disposable nappies out where you can see them. If you are wanting to wear cloth nappies then likewise, put your plastic pants, pins and nappies out in the open where you - or anyone else - can see them. Part of becoming a bedwetter is getting your head into the zone where you accept that you are already a bedwetter and the use of props to confirm that is very helpful.

Get a waterproof protector for your bed. You can get modern materials that are noiseless, but it would be better of you got a plastic one that will crinkle and make noise. It might be difficult, but if you can get an old mattress protector from another bedwetter that has already done service, it will help put your head in the 'bedwetter zone'.

A lot of people who want to be bedwetters are also adult babies and so it is a very worthwhile exercise to use this to your advantage. There are a few who are lucky enough to have an adult-sized crib or cot. Well, lucky you! Most of us are not so lucky! For the rest of us, our goal should be to infantilise our bed and make it a crib. We can do this by hanging baby toys on the bed head or similar. We can make sure we have teddy bears or dolls in our bed, knowing that they will need to be washed from time to time! Decorating the room in some kind of baby theme also helps. You might never be able to get this type of experience below, but it is worth dreaming, right?

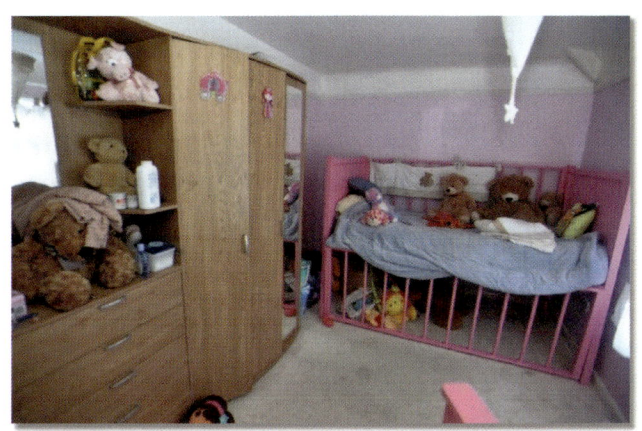

This is probably where I need to discuss the 'internal viewpoint' of your bedwetting. I am an adult baby. For me, my bedwetting is infantile. I wet the bed because I am a baby and because it is natural for someone my 'age' to do so. However, you may not be an adult baby, or you simply want your bedwetting to be 'adult bedwetting'. The practical difference is, of course, nothing at all. But in your head, you want to be a baby bedwetter or an adult bedwetter. Or perhaps both? So, decide which one makes more sense to you. To be an adult that still wets the bed or to be the baby/toddler/child that wets the bed.

And so, your scene is set, both in your mind and in your bed. So… let's wet the bed!

Overcoming negative attitudes

Let's be real here, okay? The vast majority of people think badly of bedwetting, especially in adults. The strong likelihood is that you too carry some latent bad and negative attitudes to bedwetting. We grow up being told that our wet bed is a bad thing and even that we have been disobedient and lazy. How many of us grew up being told such things? Even if our parents weren't mad about it, they certainly weren't happy and considered it a burden and let us know about it.

The attitudes that we have heard and endure often permeate our subconscious and it is there that a lot of the battle to become bedwetters again rages.

Let's start with a few positive affirmations that I want you to verbally state and approve.

Wetting the bed is okay to do

Wetting the bed is a good thing

I am allowed to wet the bed

I am proud of my wet bed (or diapers)

I want you to write these statements down and put them on your pillow during the day. I want you to say these statements out loud when you go to bed and when you wake up in the morning.

Negative attitudes to bedwetting that you hold inside you will halt your progress more than any other issue. So, say it out loud again with me right now.

Developing bedwetting

In any plan to start wetting the bed again comes the natural question of just how far you are away from it already. The reality is that some people already need to get up during the night 3-5 times to pee and even then, their pyjamas and sheets occasionally have that unmistakable odour about them. Such a person will not find it hard to slip into bedwetting – at least not minor bedwetting. Then there is the other end of the scale.

Some people are so strongly and effectively toilet trained that the chance of wetting the bed accidentally is nil, even when drunk.

These kinds of people even find it hard or difficult to pee while lying down. Fortunately, most people are in the middle.

The people who find it easiest to return to bedwetting are those that have a significant history of it while growing up. A five-year-old bedwetter is so common as to be meaningless. A ten-year-old bedwetter, however, is less common and indicates some kind of minor dysfunction either physically or emotionally. It is, however, still very common, but once you hit mid-teens, if you are still bedwetting then there is a tendency towards it that may never leave you entirely. You may indeed get night-dry, but the reasons you wet initially may still be there waiting to resurface if you give it a chance.

So, in the beginning, we need to understand and recognise the natural impediments we have to bedwetting and accept that they exist. This is what is wrong with so many 'easy' bedwetting plans in that everybody is very different. We all start at different places and so any program has to be general and take this into account.

For us, however, there is a very strong tendency to bedwetting that we need to exploit. Adult Babies seem to have a much higher rate of long-term bedwetting than the rest of the population. Statistics seem to suggest that at least 3-4 times as many ABs wet the bed well into childhood or teens than the regular population. That, therefore, gives us a head start!

First Steps

In any plan for any endeavour, the first steps are crucial. The first steps are often little more than a statement of direction and where we want to arrive at. And for that reason, I suggest that you start with a classic wet bed. Here is an example of what I mean.

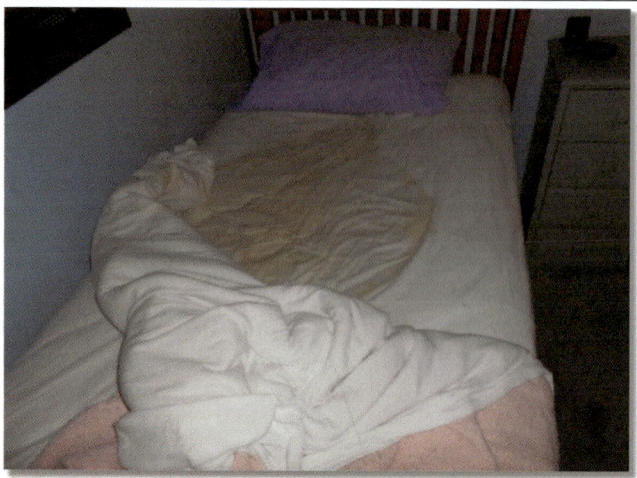

What you need to do is to get your bed looking similar to this photo. How you do it is less important than actually doing it because this is what you want to achieve. *This is your ultimate goal.*

You could just lie in bed with a full bladder and let it all empty out while you are awake and aware. It doesn't even have to be at night. You could do this during the day and then let the bed dry out leaving the damning stain of a pee-puddle.

To help get your head into the zone of becoming a bedwetter, it is helpful to actually have a wet bed there all the time as motivation and reminding you what you want. If you are not yet ready to sleep through in a wet bed then let the bed dry out before you sleep.

This is important: even if you wear diapers to bed, you should be lying on a pee-stained sheet at night, every night. The look and smell is a potent help to getting to your goal of being a bedwetter.

Now, once you accept the notion of always having a wet or stained sheet on your bed, I want to address something even more powerful. Your mattress.

Most of you will have a mattress protector, but the fact is that even with them, there is a good chance of some accidents occurring, so how about we start off giving your mattress a stain?

Just as having a stained sheet on your bed acts as a constant reminder and powerful tool towards bedwetting, so your mattress can be. And the thing about your mattress is... it is permanent. Yes, you can scrub and clean a mattress, but in large measure, if your mattress gets wet then it will stain and remain so. Therefore, just as above I want you to have a wet sheet all the time, I want you to have a wet mattress as well – or at least a dried out and stained one.

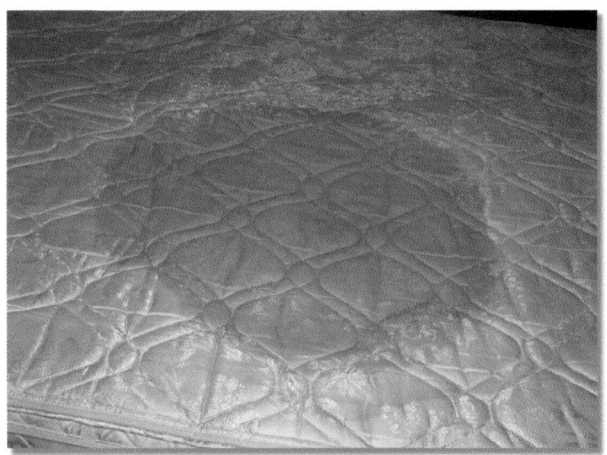

This is what your mattress needs to have – a big wet mark on it that when it dries out, leaves a stain. So, for your first deliberate wet bed, take the protector off, make sure you have a very full bladder and... let go. Let it spread everywhere, through the sheets and onto your mattress.

You don't need to do this every day or night, but you have to do it at least a few times so that your mattress gets that special and powerful look – a bedwetters mattress. It may end up looking like this:

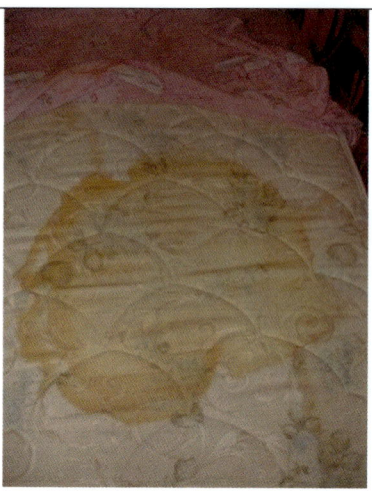

First Night

Now we are off!

The first night is exciting and bound to be a disappointment, but let's push on regardless. As described above, your bed has been prepared so that the sheets are stained, as is the mattress. Anyone who sees your bed will know that it belongs to a bedwetter and you need to tell yourself these same things.

Wetting the bed is okay to do

Wetting the bed is a good thing

I am allowed to wet the bed

I am proud of my wet bed (or diapers)

Preparing for your first night means doing all the things we were told NOT to do before going to bed as children. So, drink a lot and even some caffeinated drinks and naturally, do not use the toilet before bed.

Sleep is important and for a while, you may find falling asleep with a full bladder to be difficult. Don't worry if you can't. If you are in diapers allow yourself to pee into your diaper. Don't force it. Just let the excess flow and when it stops, let it stop even if you are not empty.

If you are undiapered, it is perhaps a little more difficult, but do the same. Just open your bladder and DO NOT FORCE IT. Just let the pee flow naturally out of you and onto the sheets.

One of the important elements is to introduce the idea of wetting being natural and unforced. So, do not force your pee out, but rather let it flow naturally and easily.

Now, diapers are warm to wear when wet, but a wet bed is not the same. In summer or warm weather, a wet bed tends to not be that uncomfortable. Indeed, most of what we think of as discomfort is nothing more than the feeling of something different to what we have experienced for so many years. After a while – and it can be a long while – a wet bed feels natural and normal and not uncomfortable at all.

What *can* help is to keep the bedroom warmer than normal. Heat your room a little more than normal and/or use a thicker quilt or blankets to make the bed warmer. That way the coldness of the wet patch won't be perceived as discomfort. A wet bed quickly warms up if you give it time.

You will wake up with probably a fullish bladder. Now you know what to do, right? You are in bed with a full bladder so what do you do? You wet the bed or diaper. This time, just force it all out onto the sheets and spend a few minutes enjoying what you have done.

Now get out of bed and take a good look at your sheets or your saggy nappy and just SMILE. You have done well! Tell yourself that!

Second and ongoing nights

The second night (or third night) might be more difficult for you. That is because the first night may have been disappointing. You may have felt uncomfortable or unable to sleep properly for a variety of reasons. You may have just been disappointed that you didn't wet in your sleep. This is when you need to get serious and just push on regardless.

Do the same as the first night by drinking heavily, saying your affirmations out loud and then going to bed knowing that you will not be using the toilet at all during the night for any reason. In the morning, empty out onto the sheets and SMILE. You are doing well.

It is important that you get into a bed that has a pee stain on it every night, even if you are in diapers. If you are wetting the sheets, you may want to wash them more regularly than you have been doing so before, but don't rush into it. Society would dictate that wet sheets should be washed, but we are rejecting that dictum right from the start. You could wash weekly or every 14 days if you want. But most importantly, when you do wash the sheets make sure that you re-wet the bed before the next night. It is an important part of the program that you are never ever sleeping in a bed without a pee stain. And don't forget the mattress. Add to those stains and make sure your statement of being a bedwetter is supported by the testimony of your mattress!

Pushing through failure

You will not become a premium bedwetter overnight. It may take a long time and I mean years and it may not, in fact, happen at all. For some, toilet training is so entrenched that we cannot totally defeat it. However, you may obtain a level of success as a deliberate or convenience bedwetter where you pee in your bed when awake and with comfort and pride. As I said before, that still makes you a bedwetter!

Determination to succeed is your most important attribute. Wet your bed every night without exceptions. Say your affirmations. Live as a bedwetter with your diapers out in the open and your wet sheets thrown back to dry and open for any and all to see. Yes, I mean it. If you want to be a bedwetter, you cannot hide it. It doesn't mean you have to flaunt it, but if you are proud of your wet sheets – and you are proud, right? – then you need to leave the sheets open. Even if no one ever sees, you need to know that they *could* be seen.

There are some conditioning ideas that may help. One is to masturbate in your wet bed/diapers exclusively. Decide that you will only ever masturbate in the wet bed and thus connect pleasure with wet beds. I know that some of you will occasionally not go through with the program and wet at night. That is wrong and harmful to your progress so as an addition to the above, I think you should deny yourself masturbation if you did not wet your bed/diaper the night before.

Having a wet bed coach

One of the powerful helps to learning to wet the bed properly is to have a coach. The best coach, of course, is a partner or someone who is as committed to the task of you becoming a bedwetter as you are. Be warned that asking your partner to be your wet bed coach is probably not going to end well, but if you are successful then here are a few suggestions on making that arrangement work.

The wet bed coach becomes more than a coach and actually drives and directs the bedwetting. The coach determines if it is nappies or sheets for night-time. The coach determines if there is to be mattress protection and how often. The coach also determines bedtimes and the amounts of fluids to be drunk.

The most important role of the coach is to literally... coach you in your bedwetting. This means that they will praise you for success and discipline you for failure. A typical discipline is a spanking for failure to wet the bed successfully or sufficiently.

The wet bed coach can be extremely powerful because training to be a bedwetter can be a lonely and singular activity. Sometimes the coach can simply be an understanding friend in whom you can confide your progress or failure and they can encourage you.

Sometimes a coach may even pee on your bed for you! But sadly, that is rare.

Becoming a bedwetter

If you are diligent, after a while you will arrive at a settled and regular standard of bedwetting that you feel comfortable with and pleased with. It may not be the premium bedwetting that you are hoping for but sometimes, progress like that can suddenly appear later on, when you aren't really trying so hard.

The above program does work, but it is totally dependent on you to work through the problems you find and to try hard every night. It is worth sharing your progress on social media sites that tolerate such things well.

In the Appendices, I have included two other programs for bedwetting that may help you find some bits of help and ideas to become the bedwetter you truly want to be.

YOU CAN BE THE BEDWETTER YOU WANT TO BE

Advanced Bedwetting

Bedwetting doesn't need to be just a basic experience of a moderate wet patch on your sheets a few nights a week. We can do MUCH better than that! Let's look at a few ideas for bedwetting beyond the basic. Let's look at Super-wet beds. Take a look at this wonderful example of letting go at night. A truly impressive bed.

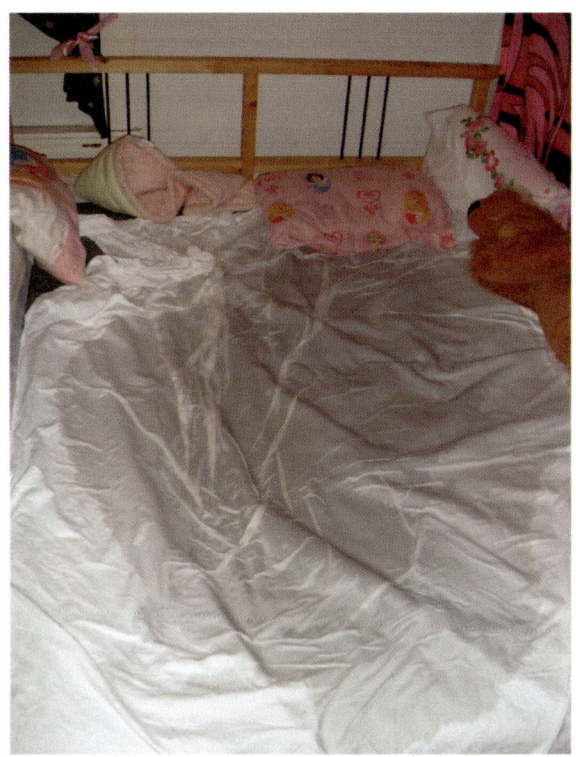

There is no need for your sheets to be merely wet. Soak them instead!

And of course, why bother with washing every night? Let those stains be your pride! Nothing like tide-lines to show off your bedwetting prowess. Multiple overlapping stains is actually part of being a bedwetter and something you will need to get used to. Make it a goal to get a well-stained sheet that is impressive. The following example is the 6th day of a bedwetting cycle. Why should yours look that much different?

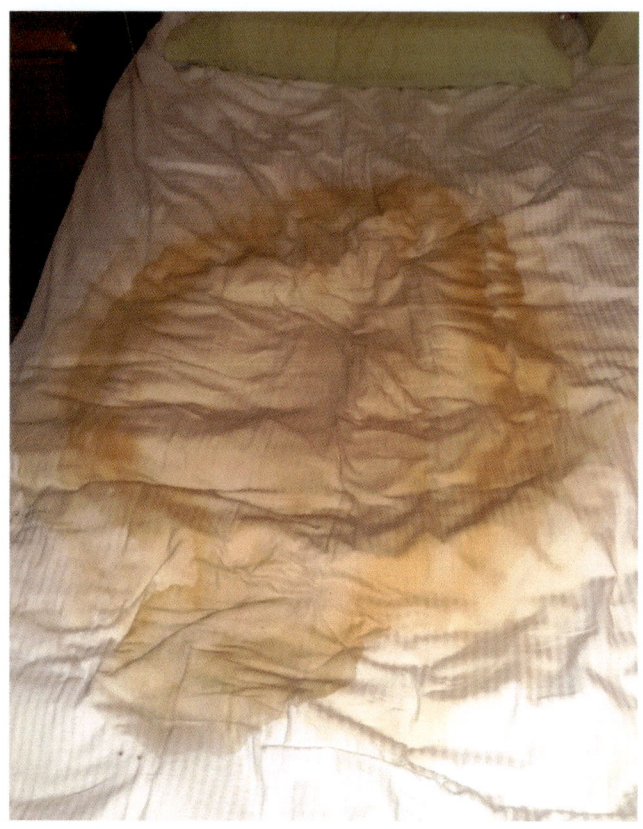

Your mattress is going to get some stains inevitably, so why not make it a point of pride and make something grand out of it? Here are some examples of stained mattresses. What do you think they say about the bedwetter that made them? Are they proud of their mattress? Pleased with their bedwetting?

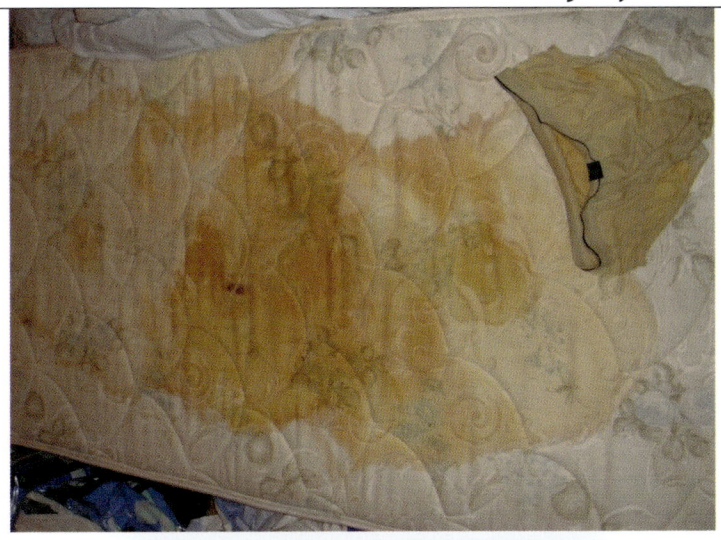

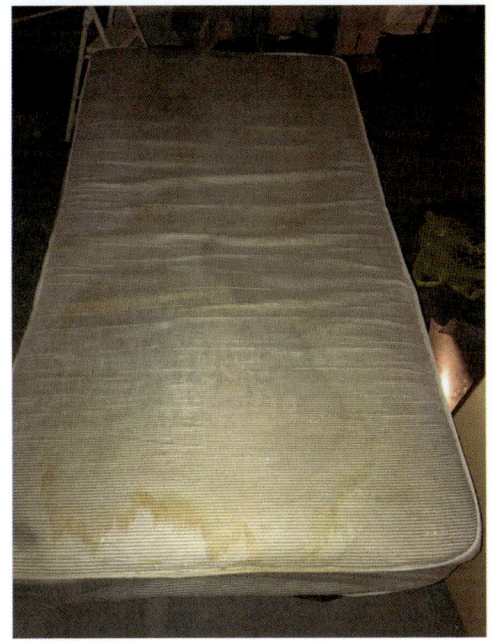

Now up until now, we have been discussing bedwetting on your own. But what about being part of a bedwetting couple where both of you wet your sheets every night? What do you think that would look like? Let's see...

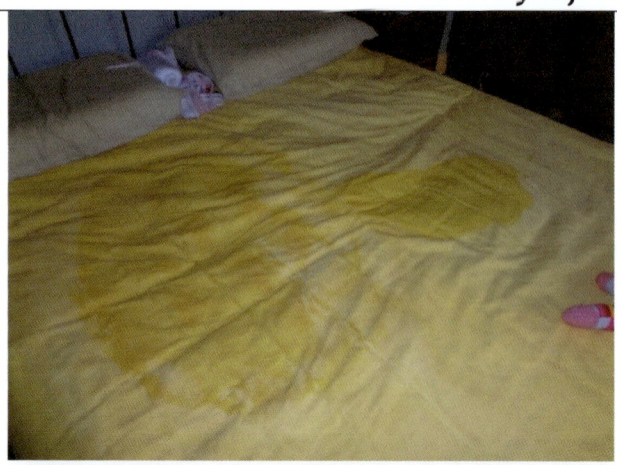

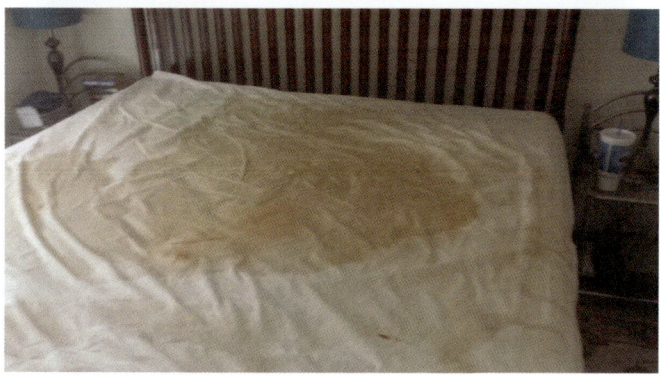

It is a truly remarkable experience to be part of a bedwetting couple and I can attest to the experience as being truly wonderful. The stigma from a wet bed is non-existent and the motivation to out-wet the other is often there. And of course, your partner is never going to hesitate to roll over in the morning for a cuddle or more because of your wetness because they are just as wet or even wetter! If you get the chance to wet with another even sporadically, do it!

Now, let me ask a question of you. Are you proud of your wet bed? Are you proud of those soaking wet diapers you have every night? Do you hide them away or do you do something radical like drying out your wet sheets outside where they can be seen? Unwashed of course, so that when they get back on the bed, they are still ready to take more wettings. Lake a look...

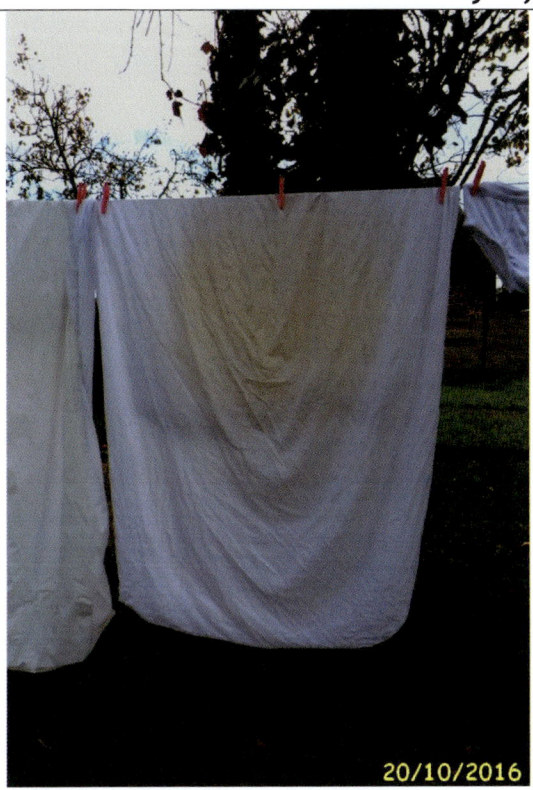

20/10/2016

Are you brave enough to do that or to dry out your pee-stained mattress in the open?

Competitive Bedwetting

There have been a few times in the past where competitions were held among bedwetters for the most impressive effort. This is judged on the size of the wet patch, mattress staining, over-flow to the side of the bed, tide-marks, pillow wetness and general colouration and artistic merit in the wet bed. Typically, the competitions are based on a portfolio of photos from day one up to as long as day 30 in the same sheets or even only as far as weekly. I have one from a competition that involved a couple's amazing wet bed effort and I show it to you now.

Perhaps it is time to revisit bedwetting competitions and a global competitive effort? Who knows!

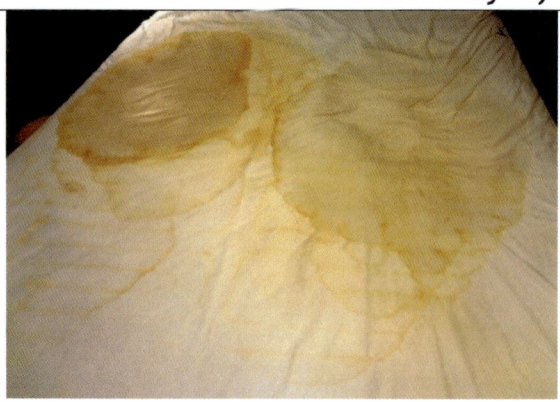

But if you want to compete as a bedwetter, the best person to compete against is yourself. Photograph your wet beds and compare them over time and see how good a bedwetter you can become. See the improvements you have been making. You don't have to share them publicly if you don't want to, but you can compete against your own best efforts quite easily and happily. Something to consider, perhaps?

Do you think you could compete in such a competition and do well? Do you think you would enjoy the competitive spirit involved in wetting as much and as creatively as you can? As I recall, there was even a prize given out – as if there needed to be much motivation to wet the bed competitively.

Wet bed pride

I have written before about how good it is to be truly proud of your wet beds, diapers and mattress. Pride helps cement bedwetting into your life and makes it easier to do and to continue. There is absolutely no reason for you to not be proud of your wet bed. You are not a child anymore wondering why your parents are angry at your wet bed and can't be proud of it like you are.

If you are proud of your wet bed, then share it with others. Take photographs and post them in places where others will see and respond to positively. Tell others how you feel about it and let them tell you how they, in turn, feel about their own wet bed. Being proud of YOUR wet bed might help another person feel good about their own bedwetting. Remember, not everyone is as confident and positive as you are about bedwetting. Some long-term bedwetters feel shame and disappointment in their wet sheets, mainly because they are conditioned to feel that way. Imagine how good it would feel if your personal wet bed pride helped another person feel good about it?

Wet bed sex

Do you feel that being a bedwetter, therefore, reduces your chances of sex? Well firstly, there is masturbation – the guy's almost-daily outlet. Do it in your wet bed. Do it face-down if you can. Do it proudly, using the wonders of your wet bed to make your masturbation longer and better and more frequent. The same applies if you use diapers at night. Masturbate in them happily and often while in bed, knowing that it is fine and good to do and that a wet bed is an ideal place to do so.

Sometimes, you may, however, be able to have sexual intercourse in your wet bed. It is easy of course if the sheets are wet and for some, may add to the eroticism to be in such an extraordinary state. What can make it interesting is if one or both of you pee on the bed some more as part of your love-making. If you are willing to try, you can form a pool of pee on the bed where one of you lies and you can get a bit of wave-motion going and a bit of splashing. Trust me... it is fun and very erotic to have wave-motion to deal with while having sex!

Golden showers are always a bit of fun and in a wet bed or a bed that is routinely peed on and stained, what difference does a little more make?

The options for enjoying good and original sex in a wet bed are many. It is, of course, dependent on your partner's acceptance of a soaking bed and that, of course, is the difficult bit. Sadly.

The issue of sheet washing

It is ironic that perhaps the single major issue with bedwetting is that of washing the sheets. Yet, despite our modern fetish for super-cleanliness, perhaps washing the sheets every night is not really necessary. In times gone by, washing of sheets was done by hand and therefore, not often. Bedwetters learned to sleep in sheets they had peed in multiple times before. Even cloth nappies were often simply hung up to dry without washing. Perhaps some of these ideas can apply to the modern happy and confident bedwetter.

In a section before I stated that if you want to become a good and effective bedwetter you should always have a sheet that has pee stains on it, even if you are wearing diapers to bed. If you wet the bedsheets themselves every night, how often do you wash them? Sadly, the answer may be the decision of someone else entirely. If you share the bed with someone else, their nose may object to the growing odour of pee and they will demand the bed be washed. Even if you don't, but you share a house with someone else, the inevitable creep of the odour into other parts of the house may also limit your endeavours. On that topic, however, you can be clever and not deliberately offend the other person and keep your windows open and your door closed and hope that the smell will be small enough to be either unnoticed or inoffensive. Be clever and inventive and not offensive to others and you should be able to keep your unwashed sheets quite a while. But you won't be able to keep them hidden and nor should you.

Wet beds need to be dried out. That's just how this works. This means that you will need to keep your quilt or blankets pulled back most of the time, so it dries off. In cooler weather, you may need to use a heater to help speed things up. One option to consider is drying off your sheets outside on a clothesline. Obviously, this is not a private thing to do as it will be noticed by other housemates, but also provides a superb drying environment. The same applies to drying out your mattress. Be warned though that a sun-warmed mattress will tend to smell strongly for some time after you bring it back in.

So how long do you wet the same sheets?

That depends on your personal preference, your situation and probably your climate. Not washing for a week is pretty basic and easy. Two weeks will also not be terribly difficult. After that, your bed will be quite smelly – although it is a delightful smell – and the stains will be getting very noticeable with multiple tide lines.

Personally, I find that it takes around ten days for a wet bed to really develop a good character, great smell and a fabulous look. After that, further nights deepen the colour and improve the feel.

Overflowing the bed

Overflowing your wet bed is a remarkable experience as it is when you wet so much and so hard that you exceed its ability to cope and it runs over the edge. Here is own of my own overflowing beds.

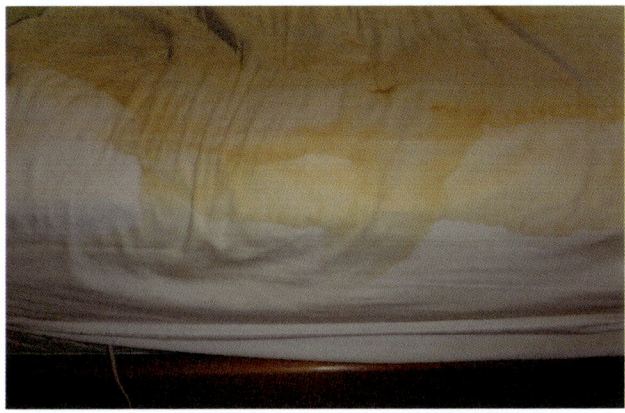

Wouldn't you feel proud in the morning to wake up and find that you had wet so much that it flowed over the edge? And the same applies to your pillow which should also start getting wet and stained.

The natural bedwetter will wet very heavily and it is inevitable that you will sometimes exceed the boundaries of your sheets and flow over the edge. Be proud of that! Let that be one of your occasional goals when you tank up before bed, hoping that your bladder will flood your bed, not merely wet it.

The question of the mattress – part two

I have written about the mattress before and it is time to face the issue head-on. Protecting your mattress is a reasonable and rational goal, but is that still okay with you? Would you not rather see your mattress deeply stained and impossible to hide your bedwetting status? Sheets and pillows can be washed. Quilts can be laundered. Rooms can be aired. But your mattress is near impossible to clean.

Your heavy bedwetting state will be obvious to you every time you make the bed or take the mattress out to be dried. Anyone who sees it will know you are not someone who had an occasional drunk accident. You are a bedwetter. A full-blown, heavy and proud bedwetter.

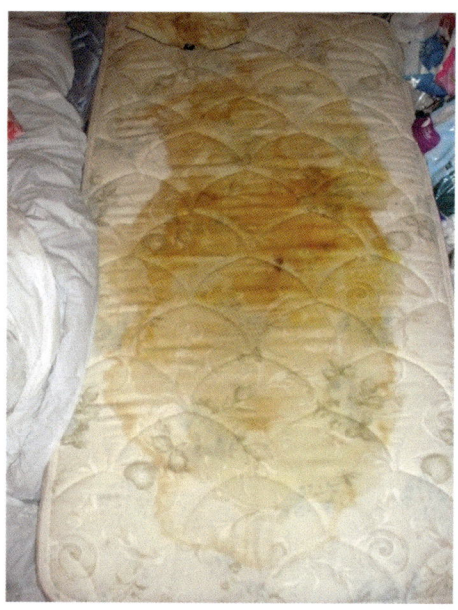

I know that having a proper bedwetter's mattress is a difficult decision to make. It means you are committing yourself to bedwetting and to the badge of honour that a super-stained mattress is. However, many serious bedwetters accept that some staining is inevitable and embrace it as part of who they are and how they wet.

You have a waterproof protector on your mattress, right? Why? I am serious here. Ask yourself why you have one on there and then consider the options. Could you perhaps occasionally take it off? Maybe a few nights a month? Maybe a night or two per week? Maybe... remove it entirely?

When I was young, I went to a friend's home who I knew was a bedwetter as it was something our parents had shared so we could do sleepovers. I did, however, see his bed without his protector - which was not very big - and his mattress was incredibly stained and it did not look that different to mine. Super-stained, super-impressive and truly wonderful. I did not know how I was feeling at the time, but I was literally really impressed with his staining. It was heavier than my own and for the first time in my life, I felt envious of his mattress. The next night at home, I took mine off the bed and soaked my mattress. This led to repeated incidents of the same thing – which did not go down well.

If you have the opportunity to regularly stain your mattress, then do so. In case you think you are alone, consider this. I used to work near a place that brought in old mattresses and I noticed that a great number of them had very obvious pee stains on them. I asked one of the pickup drivers and he told me that about two-thirds of old mattresses are peed on and a sizable number are stained hundreds of times.

If you wet your mattress occasionally, you won't even be remarkable. If you pee it hundreds of times you will be merely part of a smallish proportion.

Like I say to people, bedwetting is very, very common. No one admits to it and everyone denies it, but when they trade in their mattress, the stains are visible, and no one cares because the unstained mattress is the minority. And children's mattresses? Almost all peed on!

The Joy of Mattress-wetting perhaps?

Other bedding options

Many people use a cotton mattress protector to prevent sweat et cetera marking the mattress. Bedwetters, of course, have waterproof protectors. However, we know that when you wet in a waterproof-protected bed, the pee flows easily and far. Covering the bed and overflowing is not particularly difficult. But what about combining both?

The disadvantage is that the cotton protector tends to absorb much of the pee which makes pee-spreading harder and getting a large wet patch is more difficult. Also, drying out the bed takes much longer. The advantage, however, is that when you finally do get around to washing the sheet, you DON'T have to wash the cotton protector. That protector can stay unwashed for weeks and weeks and even longer. Then it can look like this.

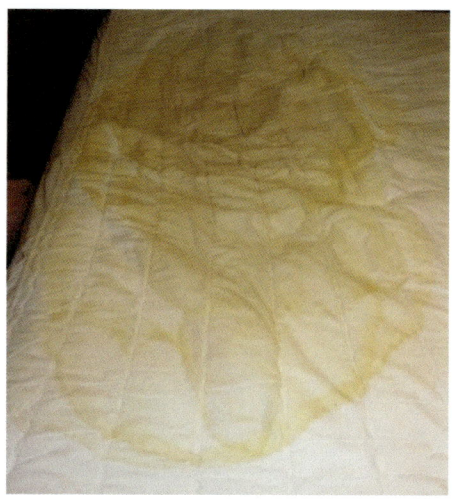

You've got to admit that this particular cotton protector looks impressive. So, if your bed-mate or housemate is demanding that you wash the sheets then you can comply, but still, have this gorgeous protector underneath. And when you wet the bed again, some of the colour and staining will rise back up.

Now, let's consider the waterproof protector itself. There are full plastic ones and some non-plastic ones, but the ones you are looking for are those that have a 'comfort liner' on top, which is basically a cotton covering so that the waterproof is not hot to sleep on. The advantage is that this cotton cover will get stained like this.

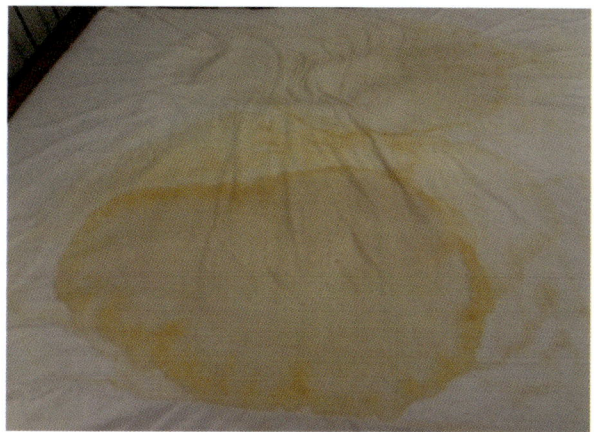

This particular example is a double-bedwetters cotton-covered waterproof and you must admit that the weeks-old tide-lines are delightful.

If you combine the cotton covered waterproof, the cotton protector and bed sheets you get this delightful soggy outcome.

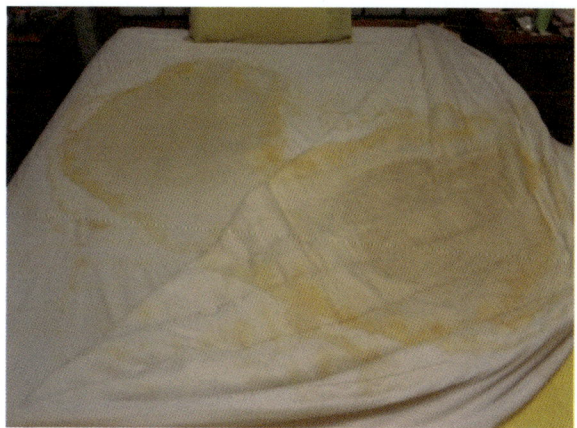

Weeks on end of practical bedwetting can result from using the right bedding.

Extra Bed-wetting

So, what do I mean by 'extra bedwetting'?

Up until now, we have talked about going to bed and peeing in there either when awake or asleep. But what about making sure that we are wetter than that? Let's be honest here. Sometimes, you will wake up and your bed will be only moderately damp, the result of a bladder that just did not comply with your wishes for a flood. It is disappointing to have put in the effort and to be rewarded with a small patch, rather than the neck to knee soaking you had hoped for. How about we give ourselves a bit more of a help?

When you pee during the day, you probably use a toilet - for those of you not in day-diapers. So why not save up your pee for night-time? You can wake up during the night and empty out and if you find it insufficient, reach for the potty next to your bed where you peed during the day and empty it into your bed! Is it truly genuine bedwetting? It is if you think it is. It is your pee and your bed and now it is wetter than before.

I've heard of people who actually pee onto their bed during the day rather than use the toilet. Okay... I have done that too. It perhaps speaks to the inner belief that some bedwetters have that the toilet is artificial and that perhaps, the bed is a better option. This is certainly an advanced and possibly rare activity, but don't dismiss it before trying it at least once.

During the day, when your bed is already peed on and you need to pee, just stand next to your bed and use it as you would a toilet. You might be surprised at just how exciting that can be.

When you work out what your own personal philosophy of bedwetting is, feel free to include any and all elements that suit you and make you feel comfortable and/or excited.

Extending the bed-as-toilet routine, we can include others. The potty you fill during the day to empty into your bed during the night or next morning doesn't need to be just your own pee. While it is relatively uncommon to have someone who will help you with this, you could every morning be lying in a bed that has additional soakings from more than just yourself! The same applies to having someone pee on your bed during the day and essentially allow them to use your bed as a pee toilet.

Sleeping wet vs sleeping dry

Up until now, we have basically assumed that you get into a dry (if stained) bed and then pee during your sleep or when you wake up, or perhaps during the night when you wake up. But that is not your only option. You can sleep in a wet bed that is already quite damp or even soaked.

To be honest, this is not everyone's cup of tea and it does take some getting used to. Also, since a wet bed tends to be cold, it is best in warm climates and in summer. However, once you get used to, it can be amazing to slip into a wet bed ready for a nap or a full night's sleep knowing that your job is not to just wet the bed, but to 'top-up' an already wet bed.

Everyone should try it before giving it away. It is best to try a nap first. Have a damp bed and then snuggle into the sheets and enjoy the unique feel of a pee-soaked bed. Perhaps add a little pee just to warm things up and then slip away for a lovely sleep.

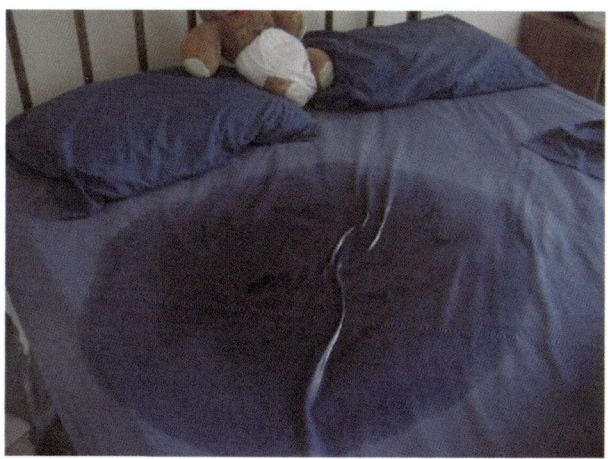

Wouldn't you like to just jump in that bed, smell the pee, feel the sense of wetness and just drift away into sleep? Hmm?

Hypnosis files for bedwetting

E veryone asks about how good these kinds of files are. Well, the news is both good and bad. Hypnosis simply does not work for everyone, but for some it does and if you are willing to persevere and are serious about it, hypnosis files really can help you achieve a better level of bedwetting.

The other issue is which ones to use. The truth is that the majority on the internet are rubbish and worthless. Hypnosis is a skill and not just a soundtrack with some words spoken. I can however highly recommend 'Charlottes' bedwetting files from baby-pants. I have used them and definitely noticed heavier bedwetting and the now absence of any dry nights at all. Other people have said similar good things.

If you are going to use them, then use them nightly and repeatedly. Don't give up after three tries. Give it a few months to teach your mind that it is okay to pee in your sleep.

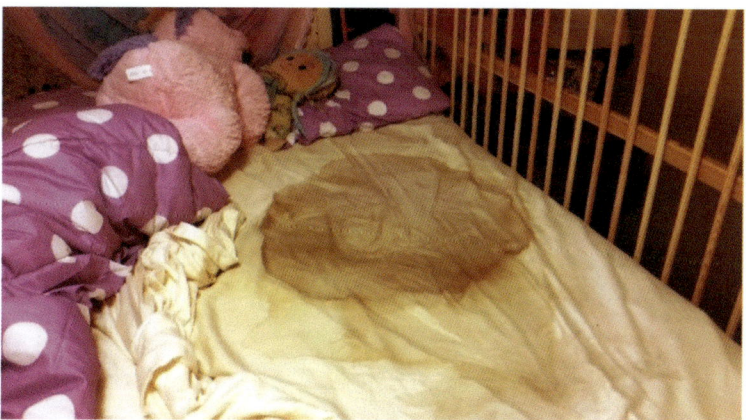

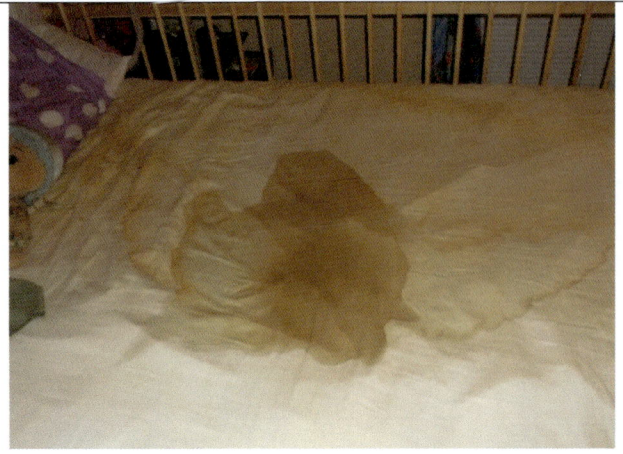

Bedwetting and ABDL

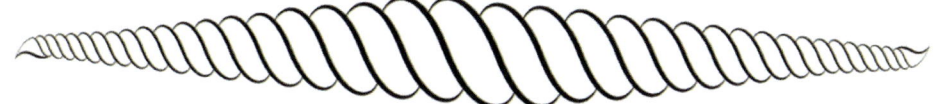

I started this book with the assumption that most readers would be ABDL although that is not necessarily true. Bedwetting is not a mere aspect of ABDL, but rather a core concern. Even if you wear diapers to bed, you will usually want genuine, premium bedwetting to occur so that you awake in a wet diaper and the great feeling of knowing that you wet your bed properly – just as a toddler or young child does every night.

The truth is that many, many ABDL want to experience some aspect of truly genuine bedwetting because it feels as if we *should* be wetting our beds still. It makes sense to us.

I know that in my own case if I am wearing a night nappy, I feel devastated if I wake and it is still dry. If I am not wearing a nappy, I am always disappointed if the sheets are anything less than awash. Even a tiny damp patch disappoints me. I am an adult baby and less than proper bedwetting disturbs me. Despite my bedwetting heritage, I took a long time to really refine and develop my bedwetting to the state it is today where I have no more than a single night per year when I am not wet. And I hope to eliminate that as well.

Incontinence and the bedwetter

Bedwetting is a form of incontinence as we all know. However, for what we are doing, it is still controlled in that it occurs in a safe place at a predictable time and it is bounded, literally by our bedding. But do we want to go further and take our bedwetting out of the bedroom and into our days? I know I did and chose the path that leads me to being in day diapers all the time now and not regretting it for a single moment. It is wonderful, exhilarating and fits perfectly with my philosophy of bedwetting and being a baby.

As you embrace bedwetting yourself, you will probably hope to achieve premium bedwetting, where you go to sleep and during the night your body naturally wets the bed without waking you. It may take some time, but it is both natural and desirable. After that, you may want to take your bedwetting with you in the form of day incontinence and diapers. I will not dissuade you. Personally, I think this is the next obvious step and in today's diaper world, pretty easy to do.

But for now, I wish you all the success you want as you seek to wet your beds happily and successfully. I hope this book has helped to encourage and motivate you as well as give you a few hints on how to go about it.

Stay wet and stay happy!

Appendix One: Bedwetting Research

In 2002 one enterprising bedding company developed a non-plastic mattress protector for bedwetting children. The sales were quite good, but feedback from retailers was that a surprisingly high number of customers were discreetly asking if they were available in Double and Queen-bed sizes. When the company first produced them, the demand was so high that it exceeded production levels for over six months. According to the company, adult waterproof covers are now over 40% of their sales and still growing. That was the clue that bedwetting was far more prevalent than previously thought. Their experience was no surprise to some, however.

Kirste and Franklin (1991) researched the level of bedwetting in all strata of society and quickly realised that it was far, far higher than previously thought. When defined as one wet bed a week the figures for bedwetting were as follows:

Age	Percentage that wet the bed (once a week)
5	72.2
6	69.7
7	55.1
8	42.1
9	28.9
10	17.2
11	11.4

12	10.5
13	8.5
14	7.8
15	6.1
15-20	6.2
20-30	5.6
30-40	12.6
40-50	13.9
50-60	28.2
60-70	30.1
70-80	41.6
80+	51.9

This report shocked and surprised most doctors and educators who at first refused to believe that bedwetting was so prevalent. It was soon discovered that there was more shame in bedwetting than in sexual abuse, incest or severe mental illness. For centuries, bedwetting had been under-reported by as much as two orders or magnitude. This same report also went on to identify the frequency of *problem bedwetting* and defining it as 5-7 times a week. The results were equally surprising.

Age	Percentage that wet the bed (5-7 times/week
5	41.2
6	36.3
7	30.2
8	20.3
9	19.4

10	12.5
11	9.6
12	9.3
13	6.5
14	5.1
15	4.6
15-20	4.9
20-30	1.9
30-40	5.2
40-50	8.6
50-60	6.0
60-70	9.8
70-80	13.9
80+	19.9

The oft-quoted statement that adult bedwetting affects about 1% of the community was based on just one target group, those in their peak physical period of ages 20-30. For everyone else, bedwetting was more than just common, it was *very* common.

This same study researched sibling relationships with bedwetting prevalence. The summarised results stated that:

"If one child over 8 years of age was wetting the bed three times a week or more, the chance of another sibling being an atypical [over age of 8] bedwetter was approximately double (1.86 factor) that of the single-child average. Likewise, the presence of two atypical bedwetting siblings makes the third child 2.72 times as likely to be a bedwetter. With three atypical bedwetters, the fourth child has a significantly higher 7.9 times average chance while with four existing bedwetters, the fifth child has 42 times average likelihood. While statistically invalid due to small sample

*numbers, there was no single example of a sixth (or higher)
sibling being a non-bedwetter if the other five were."*

It is clear that bedwetting has a strong family link both from
parents and siblings. Parental bedwetting history was obviously a
factor and Kirste stated:

*"If one parent was a bedwetter until at least age 20, the
likelihood of a child being a bedwetter increased by
approximately 25%, which is considered to be a relatively small
change. However, if both parents were bedwetters, the chance
rises dramatically to around 950% higher, thus making a child of
dual bedwetting parents almost a certainty to have some level of
bedwetting."*

Kirste then made the astonishing statement that has been
criticised widely, but not repudiated.

*"Parental attitudes to bedwetting and particularly the wet bed
itself seems to be of great significance in the extinguishing of
bedwetting in ages 5-20. Condemnatory and abusive attitudes by
parents have historically been shown to be totally ineffective in
the incidence of pre-teen bedwetting and lead mainly to secretive
behaviour and lowered self-image and often delays the
extinguishing of bedwetting instead. Parents with an accepting
and compassionate response to childhood bedwetting do appear
to have a moderate influence on reducing bedwetting although it
appears to be quite small and very unpredictable. A third
category of parents form a part of a hitherto unknown subset
that can be best described as 'attitude neutral' to the issue of
bedwetting."*

Early in our interviews, we discovered this third category in
answers to the question of 'when do you think your child will stop
bedwetting?' Classically the expected answer would be 'When he/she
matures' or 'When he/she is ready', meaning physically ready. The
surprise answers to this also included the following:

- He will stop when he decides it is no longer appropriate

- I would never make my child stop. It is up to him to choose to or not [emphasis mine]
- There is nothing wrong with bedwetting!
- It isn't a priority for us to be concerned about bedwetting (from a parent of a 16-year-old girl)

There were a variety of like responses, but can be best summarised by describing them as parents who are not concerned at their child's bedwetting and do not consider it a negative behaviour or a priority. There were also small numbers who considered bedwetting in almost praise-worthy terms. It was noted that families where both parents were heavy bedwetters, tended to not make as much effort to end their children's bedwetting and in a number of cases actively promoted it as a positive experience.

In response to his discovery, we researched attitudes to bedwetting among existing bedwetting parents. Our initial findings showed nothing unexpected in single bedwetting parents, but where both were bedwetters, the answers were indeed surprising. Out of 13000+ original respondents, the dual-parental bedwetter group comprised 696 couples.

Do you find your own bedwetting experience?

Very negative 6.2%

Negative   29.1%

No concern   51.2%

Positive   13.5%

What surprised everyone was the shocking discovery that the underlying assumption that bedwetting was a bad and negative experience for all wetters was simply not completely true. There were not only some, but a surprisingly high number of people, for whom bedwetting was at worse of no concern and then some that actually felt it was *positive*. A number of researchers followed up on this and studied individual attitudes to their own bedwetting. The previous assumption that it was a negative behaviour needed some reinvention.

Sykes in 1995 studied 975 adult bedwetters ranging from 18 to 55 years. He explains the age choice as trying to exclude both old-age bedwetting and child/adolescent bedwetting and to focus on 'atypical' bedwetters, although previous studies would suggest that 'atypical' was the wrong choice of word. His first survey dealt with the frequency of wet beds starting with once a month. He also noted that 'bedwetter' included the category of people who wore nappies to bed and that while the bed itself was still dry, bedwetting was still occurring.

Frequency of Bedwetting	Percentage
Once a month	15.1
Twice a month	6.5
Once a week	10.6
2 times a week	6.5
3 times a week	12.4
4 times a week	4.3
5 times a week	8.4
6 times a week	6.3
7 times a week	3.9

His survey did, however, demonstrate that despite the belief that the frequency of adult bedwetting incidents in sufferers was low, almost a quarter (22.9%) wet the bed more than half the time and one in 25 wet every night.

He was the first to tread into the truly treacherous area of whether or not bedwetting had a component of *choice* or more accurately, was *deliberate*. The generally accepted belief is that no one deliberately wets the bed. It is also an article of faith that no child deliberately wets the bed and yet we have categories of mental disorders in children that have them doing exactly that. Sykes discovered that there was a small, but significant sub-grouping that wet the bed either by choice or without exerting any appreciable effort to cease. Surprisingly aware of the 'diaper fetish' crowd, Sykes excluded fetishists from his group using control questionnaires. Of peripheral interest was that this excluded only 19 people and did not materially affect any previous or subsequent results.

304 (31.8%) people stated that they took no practical steps at all to stop their bedwetting (as opposed to wear protection or seeking medical intervention) and the surprisingly high figure of 98 (9.9%) people stated that they 'deliberately wet their bed at times'.

The follow-up question addressed the frequency of deliberate bedwetting.

Frequency of Deliberate Bedwetting	Percentage
Rarely	25.5%
Sometimes	15.3%
Often	11.4%
Weekly	4.2%
Twice weekly	6.2%
Nightly	5.3%

Again, he looked for the link between deliberate bedwetting and parental influence. The results were not surprising really.

"The numbers of respondents who deliberately wet their beds once a week or more had a very high incidence of dual-parent bedwetters (67%). Those with a deliberate bedwetting incidence of less than once a week showed little correlation to parental bedwetting or influence.

Common reasons given were:

It is comfortable/comforting

It makes me feel safe

It makes me feel proud

Although the numbers were small, it should be noted that deliberate bedwetters of a frequency of more than once a week also tended towards reduced sheet changes. A typical response was changing wet sheets between 2 and 3 weeks. Those deliberate bedwetters who wore nappies as a rule also tended to have unprotected nights without nappies.

An unstudied further aspect was the prevalence of unprotected mattresses. Of 98 deliberate bedwetters, 11 did not use waterproof protection and comments indicated an accumulated pride on the development of staining patterns. This was also evident in protected mattresses when there was anecdotal commentary on a pride of overlapping and multiple urine stains on bedding and pillows.

The discovery of significant levels of bedwetting that was not accidental and did not carry stigma or embarrassment then led one researcher to ask the question no one had even conceived of prior to this. If we extrapolate the adult results, we can assume with some level of confidence that some children also deliberately wet the bed. Naturally, the question is to ask why they would do so. The difficulty in obtaining reliable quantities of deliberate bedwetting children led the researcher to speculate to a large degree, but the results were still significant.

Some of these dual bedwetting parents even punished dry beds and sent the child back to wet the bed in the morning. One such child when married was still unable to feel comfortable in dry sheets and frequently wet the sheets before going to bed and co-opted his wife to assist.

Hite refers to an unspecified 1960s medical report that identified that some children and teens were unaware that bedwetting was not socially acceptable and the major reason they still bedwet was the absence of a genuine reason or motivation. In trying to find a reason for this Hite dismissed intellectual disability which was the common explanation at the time. She came up with two possible reasons. One was that the child was raised in a house that did not stigmatise or even seek to correct bedwetting (or pants wetting) and therefore grew up with little experiential understanding of negative social impacts. This was particularly strong in families where most or all members remained bedwetters. The second reason was one that appears to link closely to the modern paraphilia of infantilism or Adult Babies.

> *"A small number of respondents appear to have matured in most normal developmental areas, but with some personality and behavioural segments remaining strongly linked to the infantile stage and remaining there even well into adulthood. Despite more than adequate intelligence, the rationale of stopping bedwetting or even pants-wetting does not seem to find traction in their minds. It is as if cognitive reasoning in a small number of segments remains locked at the infantile stage of development. Therefore, because their view and control over continence remains at this infantile level, toilet training and bedwetting, in particular, develops slowly, late or not at all. This is explainable in part because the child does not make the connection between their biological age and their continence development. They are neither unable nor unwilling to be dry. They just haven't fully developed emotionally where it is yet important enough to be acted on.*

Such children are often described wrongly as deliberate bedwetters or pants wetters (or soilers, as the same applies), but this is quite wrong. They are in still operating at the infantile level where wetting and soiling without control or negative effect is acceptable and the default state. Such people struggle to find a reason to stop because if the practical aspects of bedwetting are handled (nappies or exemplary hygiene etc) the motivation to stop simply does not exist from an internal perspective. There has to be external reasoning involved. This may be pressure from family, partners and friends, but one respondent explained that he stopped his bedwetting because of his wife, but even now some twenty years later, he doesn't understand why he had to and as a result, still has significant relapses.

Anecdotal evidence suggests that some of these children and adolescents express some of this incomplete development through infantilism [adult babies] and other regressive behaviours."

Summary:

Bedwetting is not at all what we think it is and probably never has been. The polite society notion of 99.9% of children being night-dry by age 8 is a fallacy. Even the idea of all adults remaining dry until the onset of very old age is likewise an unsupported fantasy. Not only that, the levels of bedwetting are huge and vastly more than previously believed. However, it is still not a topic of easy discussion as most bedwetters fear the response, especially from often clueless medical professionals. And all of this is before we even think about bedwetters who do so without concern or who actively choose to sleep wet.

In the middle of this is the growth in the numbers of children who are bedwetting longer and with less concern. Many parents are delaying general toilet training until pre-school begins and often only for that reason.

One mother posted on a parenting blog only a few months ago, that indicates just how more open we are now and how better we are getting informed on the not-so-secret (and not-so-new) phenomenon of bedwetting.

"...My son had his four friends over for a sleepover just last month. They were all thirteen and as silly as boys that age typically are. But what shocked me most were the phone calls from three of their mothers to inform me that their son wets the bed. At 13! Now those who know me can giggle as my hypocrisy is now in full flight. My own son had only stopped his bedwetting six months earlier and that was the reason he was having his first-ever sleepover in the first place. We hadn't even removed his waterproof sheet from the bed yet as I was not yet convinced of

his permanent dryness. His father is still a bedwetter from time to time so I had natural scepticism. [Note: 'time to time' is a euphemism for dry sometimes!] Sigh...

I felt quite intimidated by the prospect of three wet beds in the morning, none of them from my own family. But what I couldn't fathom was the boys wanting to risk almost certain discovery. I had wet my own bed until nine so I knew the drama intimately and I was mortified if even my mother found out, never-mind my friends.

The morning after the sleepover, I was standing just outside the bedroom door wondering how to discreetly enter and afford each boy the chance to get out of his probably wet bed undiscovered. Then I listened to them talking and laughing and even giggling like girls. They were comparing each other's wet bed! Serious!! They were discussing whose was the BEST wet bed, meaning the biggest. I couldn't hear much detail and so walked away in a daze and called to them from the kitchen to get up and get some food.

Ten lazy minutes later, all five boys wandered into the kitchen and four of them had obviously wet pyjamas on! Including my son! No-one gave a shit that they were wet. It was as if it were the most natural thing in the world to them. I was aghast, but I was the only one. My husband got up soon after and was equally surprised to see (and smell) four wet boys. He had wet the bed as well, but unlike the boys, I make him shower before even leaving the bedroom if he has wet.

Together we went to my son's bedroom and saw four enormous wet, soaking beds.

This has blown me away and even more so because my son has not been dry since and my efforts to discuss it with him have been fruitless. He simply doesn't care.

I had two phone calls that morning from mothers asking me how it had gone and when I mentioned that all but one had wet the bed, they seemed relieved that their son was not being singled out. Being the tactless woman some of you know, I asked one if bedwetting ran in the family and the silence was deafening on the other end. When I admitted (rather stupidly) that my husband still wet the bed, she literally whistled a sigh and admitted that both she and her husband were bedwetters as well. I heard far more from her than I ever wanted to know. It was if I had opened a floodgate (bad pun, I know). Apparently, they both wet the bed every night (do I really need to know that?) and their three children also wet the bed – also every night.

It was the tone in her voice that disturbed me more than the words. She seemed excited to tell me and not the least bit embarrassed. And she has been pestering me to go over there for dinner and part of me wants to and the other part terrified. I would be the only adult at the table that doesn't wet the bed and it would appear the only one who has a problem with it. The children's table would likewise have only one non-bedwetter as well which is my daughter. I now classify my son as a bedwetter again.

Did I miss the memo? When did bedwetting become the new minority movement?

Thoughts anyone?"

Appendix Two: Thoughts on bedwetting for parents and partners

T his article was found on the internet and is relevant to this discussion.

This document is written for open-minded parents/partners of child, teen and adult bedwetters. It puts a different slant on the common issue of bedwetting and why it may not be a problem at all and may, in fact, be a life choice. And this applies equally to your bedwetting partner.

First Points...

One of the embarrassing aspects of being a young child is the ever-present fact of bedwetting. The parent is perhaps ashamed, and the child is confused and frustrated. Well, that is probably true for the majority, but the surprising truth is that it is only the majority opinion. A few children will wet the bed with no real idea that it is 'wrong' or that they can stop if they want to. They don't want to stop wetting the bed and in their immature minds, they question WHY they should stop. The notion of a dry bed is foreign and the motivation to be dry is small or non-existent. And in the background, just may stand a parent looking on and secretly wishing for a wet bed just as they wet the bed as children and perhaps, still do.

Frequency of Bedwetting:

The internet has been a great equaliser and breaker of false information and so, it has been with bedwetting. Historically, bedwetting has been the domain of young children and the elderly and something not to be spoken of... at all. But today, we are aware of a much different story and while the rest of the world believes the myth that bedwetting over age of five is uncommon and in teenagers and adults, quite rare, we know differently.

Bedwetting is commonplace. Adults, teens, children... all wet the bed.

Bedwetting Myths:

Bedwetting is never deliberate. One of the worst bits of advice ever given by professionals to parents is that kids <u>never</u> deliberately wet the bed. Children *do* deliberately wet the bed. Sometimes, it will be passive deliberation by not taking any steps to stop it. Other times it will be active deliberate bedwetting where the child or teen will pee their bed fully awake and then sleep in it. While it might be relatively uncommon, it is far from rare. No one has explained to them why they should stop wetting the bed... so they don't. It is the same with teens and adults. The idea that it is always accidental should be dismissed and accept that it *may* be deliberate. The underlying assumption by parents and professionals alike is that bedwetting is so *obviously* wrong that any child teen or adults will work hard to end it. It is generally true, but not all the time.

In a family situation that keeps the child in diapers until bedwetting ends, the comfortable diaper takes away any of the discomfort and instead relies on peer-pressure, parental pressure or internal motivations to stop. But what if none of those exist? What if the child never understands *or cares* that bedwetting is 'wrong'? If natural physical development does not intervene and over-ride, bedwetting may not end quickly, or at all.

Bedwetting is uncomfortable. A soaking wet bed certainly *can* be uncomfortable for many and probably most, but for some, it is not only not UNcomfortable, some find it a *comfort* to sleep in a wet bed. Parents or spouses operating on the assumption that the wet bed is highly uncomfortable may be surprised at why their child or partner seems upset that the sheet is changed during the night when they are quite happily lying in it. For some children, teens and even adults, the wet bed is the preferred sleeping mode at times. A partner may be frustrated that their bedwetting partner seems oblivious to it and prefers to have wet sheets without washing.

In warm weather, a wet bed may be quite fine and comfortable. Even in cooler weather, a warm house may also make a wet bed quite okay to sleep in.

The point is this: assuming that a wet bed is uncomfortable is only partly reasonable. It may in fact, not be so.

Bedwetting is a shame. For young children and adults, bedwetting isn't a shame at all and anyone that makes it so, do them a disservice. For older kids, teens and adults, it is assumed that a wet bed is an object of great shame and for many, that is undoubtedly so. For a significant number, however, (and a growing number), bedwetting is an object of pride and achievement. Rather than a failure, it is considered an accomplishment. You don't have to understand it for it to be true!

Shaming your children, your partner, your friend or even yourself for bed-wetting is a very bad thing to do. Even if you are trying to help them stop wetting their bed, making them feel ashamed will absolutely never work. In fact, it will probably make things worse as well as make them feel bad toward you.

Bedwetting is 'bad'. The idea that a minority behaviour is 'bad' is appalling. We need to have better rationales than that. There is nothing inherently 'bad' about bedwetting. Certainly, it is a minority that wet the bed, but it is far from a small number that do so. Wetting in your sleep in your bed or even while awake is far from a terrible thing. It may be unavoidable, or it may be a choice or it may simply be something you don't care about at all. Wet or dry, it is just sleeping!

Bedwetting ruins relationships. Truth is, bedwetting *can* damage relationships, but at the same time, so can a great deal of other things. Anecdotal evidence suggests that bedwetting is an inconvenience in a relationship rather than a killer, and that is assuming that only one wets the bed. There are a growing number of couples that both wet the bed and rather than cause conflict, it is a point of commonality.

Is my child or partner wetting the bed deliberately?

It is a very complex question because it is not necessarily a yes/no answer. They may just have not found a reason to stop or they may have decided bedwetting is for them.

Sometimes looking at your child or teen (or adult) with wider eyes can answer the question for you. Do they take any steps to *not* wet the bed eg getting up during the night, fluid reduction before bed etc? Or do you see the opposite behaviour - loading up on drinks and not using the toilet before bed. This is deliberate bedwetting. How could it be anything else?

Say for example that you have a healthy 16-year-old boy, plays sports and is active with friends, yet wets his bed solidly every night. The question isn't *is* he deliberately wetting the bed, because he clearly is. This is the bit of thinking you need to understand now. If your teenager is wetting the bed every night yet is totally healthy, what are the chances it is completely accidental? The perhaps unpleasant truth is that you *may* have a deliberate bedwetter. The question now is 'what do I do about it?'

What do I do about my deliberate bedwetter?

The first issue is why you think you should do *anything at all* about it. Parents often feel the need to 'do something' about issues they feel are important and sometimes that is the wrong decision. Your child *wants* to wet their bed and you should respect and honour that. Let them wet their bed, but it is fair to establish rules about it. It is, however, totally unfair to expect them to *stop* wetting the bed. Can you honestly establish a rational explanation as to why a wet bed is an unacceptable life choice? Sure, it is problematic and extra work, but that is not the same as wrong or unacceptable. It is just a life-choice to remain a bedwetter. It is a choice they may change later on and most likely will, but for now, let it be.

Discuss the bedwetting with them and explore with them their decision to wet the bed. Be supportive of their wetting and understand that it is deeply important to them. Sheet changing is very important and you probably don't understand this: stained sheets are a goal, not a problem. Because of this, they will most likely resist you on washing the sheets. Look at it like this: you get less workload from weekly sheet washing instead of daily washing and they get all they want as well, which is in part, an obviously wet bed.

The question is often asked about the damage to the bedwetter's mattress. While plastic waterproofs will completely protect a mattress, it is remarkably often that these sheets get 'damaged' or mysteriously removed, causing massive staining to the mattress. If this is already happening to your bedwetter, you will need to address this as a mutual responsibility. Your child wants a stained mattress because you won't be washing away the evidence of their wetting. It is permanent, cumulative and a constant reminder of their bedwetting. This is a difficult one because it has practical difficulties. Soaking wet mattresses are a problem unless it is managed right and that is your challenge - not to forbid, but to manage. If you can air-dry the mattress once a week then it will be more than fine. Once a month is a minimum. Drying in direct sunlight works well, but it also creates a smelly mattress for a few hours. Decide with your bedwetter if you and he wants the smelly mattress option because your bedwetter probably finds the smell intoxicating. Ensuring a regularly dried mattress allows you and your bedwetter to maintain constant communication over the topic and therefore to address issues and changes.

What about nappies?

Most deliberate bedwetters will involve nappies at some stage and that may be confusing for you. They may wear nappies to bed at night and keep the sheets dry or they may start wearing nappies during the day to retain the pleasure of wetness outside the bed. They may also want both wet sheets and nappies which is a difficulty as you can imagine.

Nappies are an inevitable experience for the deliberate bedwetter. They will wear them and experiment with how they fit into their lives. As they get older, they may have the need to occasionally be dry at night, but without much experience in dryness the nappy is employed to ensure it. They may also choose to wear nappies during the day, and this could be done to promote daytime wetting.

Appendix three: How to Become a Bedwetter

One of the most exciting things that can happen to a person is to wake up wet from head to toe, or with soaking diapers - the result of yet another embarrassing' night-time accident. Do you do that - or would you like to?

Unfortunately, it's not as easy as just 'wanting to', as it takes a lot of practice and commitment. There are some seemingly 'magical' methods like subliminal hypnosis tapes, but the jury is still out on how well they work.

The following is really just a guide to start you off and depending on how far you want to go, you can build on it with your own ideas.

First, you must prepare your bed. Get a strong plastic mattress cover because you are going to need it. If you can get an old pee-stained mattress that would be better, as it would be a good visual reminder of your aim. But by the end of your training even your good mattress will have stains on it!

You are now a bedwetter! Don't forget that! Your nights will now involve soaking sheets, panties, pajamas, and diapers. What you will need at this point is commitment to the goal of being a real bedwetter. Even when you may not want to wet the bed you must. When friends stay over or you visit them, a wet bed or diapers will result every morning! You will have to explain to several people why you still wet your bed and that reason is that you have always wet your bed! Probably the most important factor in becoming a bedwetter is to think of yourself as one, and having other people know about your bedwetting is very important to helping you along the trail.

Phase One:

On the very first wet night, you should sleep in an unprotected bed – no plastic sheet and no diapers! Your mattress will suffer, but that is what bedwetting is all about. On the following nights use a plastic sheet, although remember that you should occasionally sleep in an unprotected bed. As it dries outside many people will see all the bedwetter stains on it.

For four hours before going to bed you are to drink heavily, and no going to the toilet. When you go to bed just try to go to sleep despite the pressure of a full bladder. You will probably wake up in a few hours, and when you do, first of all, you must empty your bladder there and then. Just let yourself wet deliberately and completely empty your bladder and begin to enjoy your first wet bed! If you awake a few times wet even more. You need to get used to the idea of wetting in a bed. It can take some time to get over toilet training where we were all expected to be good and get up to go in the toilet, but the bed is a better place!

While you are wetting, enjoy all the sensations of the warm flow soaking all around you. If you are a girl, concentrate on the delightful feeling of pee soaking down between your legs and under your bum, or if you are a guy, you can have the added joy of aiming the stream up over your stomach and letting it flow off the sides and down into the sheet. After you have finished, make sure you masturbate in your wet sheets and pajamas. This way you will associate even more pleasure with bedwetting, and you should avoid masturbating anywhere else other than in your wet sheets or later, your wet diaper.

In the morning you should spend 30 minutes just lying in and wriggling about in your wetness. When you get up, inspect the damage to your bed. See how big the wet stain is on your mattress. Enjoy the naughtiness of what you've done! You are on the way to becoming a real bedwetter! On the first night you will need to dry out your mattress. If possible, put it outside where others may see it - your neighbours or anyone who comes over.

Although it may take some effort at first to wet your bed, eventually it will become easier. Continue following this same procedure every night until you find that wetting in your bed is easy and natural, even if it is still totally deliberate. This may take several weeks but you must feel relaxed and comfortable wetting in your bed. The important thing is to make sure you wet every time you wake up, even if it's only a little bit. After a while, you will only half wake up, just long enough to have an 'accident' and then go back to sleep.

Phase Two:

You should be comfortably wetting your bed deliberately every night and should have no difficulty in doing so. Now we are going to introduce full-night bedwetting and diapers. You are going to sleep wet all night! Same rules - no drinking for at least 4 hours or even more. The point is that you must have a full to bursting bladder when you go to bed. Go to bed at least an hour earlier so you can spend your time doing this and enjoying it, but first of all, you must get your diapers and plastic pants on.

Before you get into bed, make a big deal about having to wear diapers. Tell yourself the reason you need them and enjoy all the sensations of putting them on. If you can involve your partner, so much the better. Savour the feel and texture of the diapers, the smell of the plastic pants and baby powder, the pressure and bulky feeling between your legs, and the feel of the pants sliding up your legs. Stand and look at yourself in the mirror and remember that you're dressed like that because you are a naughty bedwetter.

Jump into bed, and as soon as the light is out, relax and wet your diapers completely. Revel in the warmth as it spreads out around your middle. Now you are going to have to sleep in them all night - no excuses! Once again spend some time enjoying yourself - slip your hand down inside the warm diaper and make yourself come. Girls might enjoy rolling onto their fronts and rocking back and forwards on the bulky pad. When you wake up during the night you must continue to wet immediately even if there isn't much there.

If you have visitors or are sleeping over, you're going to have to explain about your bedwetting. This can actually be quite good fun. Tell them that you wet the bed beforehand so you can put your plastic sheet on, but after everyone has gone to bed, be the naughty bedwetter you're expected to be. If the opportunity arises, even let them see your bed with the wet sheets still on it.

Phase Three:

By this stage, it should be feeling almost natural to be wet. You need to get to the point where you truly feel comfortable with being wet all night, can wet very easily lying down in bed and are able to do it first thing upon waking up. The purpose of all this is to unlearn the idea that having a wet bed or diapers is uncomfortable. By now you should really be looking forward to being wet and enjoying it. Repeated deliberate bedwetting, especially in a half-waking state, will also get your brain used to associating the idea that 'it's alright to wet the bed' with the pressure you feel in your bladder.

What happens from now on depends totally on getting your mind used to the idea that wetting the bed is OK, and on how committed to this goal you are.

If you can keep trying, eventually you will succeed.

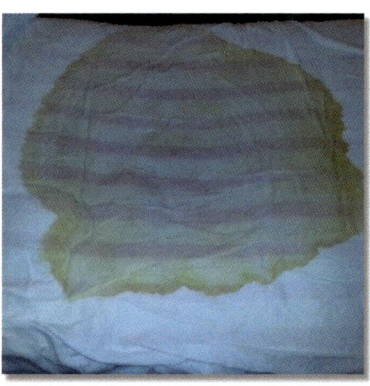

Appendix four: The Bedwetting Trainee

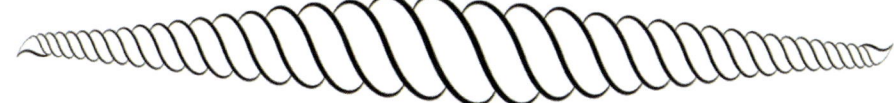

Materials Required:

Diapers, cloth or disposable, mattress covers, clock with multiple alarm settings, child's wetting calendar.

Preparation - the week before training begins:

1st the trainee must understand that from the start of training they are to be considered a bedwetter in every sense of the word. The term "Nocturnal Enuresis" should be readily available if a nurse or doctor asks if the trainee has a medical condition. They do have a medical condition, and they should understand that now before the training really begins. This needs to be understood in all its permutations: there will be no place the trainee won't be able to wet, they will have to wear protection every night. There will be embarrassing questions, and staying over with friends, and dating will be forever changed by this behavior.

2nd the trainee should start going to bed at an early time. 10 pm would be ideal, but as late as 11 pm works. If the trainee works on a specific schedule adjust times so that they should get at least 8 hours of sleep nightly. They should also get in the habit of having a drink before bed.

3rd the trainee should begin sleeping in the diapers that they will be wearing most through the training. Cloth diapers are recommended. They should be comfortable sleeping in the diaper, and should practice wetting while lying in bed, finding the most comfortable positions to do so.

4th the trainee should be prepared to be honest about their wetting. There will be some aspects of the later phases where the trainee will have to self-report how their night went, and the only way to establish the proper behavior is if the trainee reports honestly.

Phase 1 - The New Behavior Paradigm - 1 month duration

Take the clock and set three alarms for 1 AM, 2 AM and 3 AM. These times are important because it allows the trainee to get a solid amount of sleep, but not enough for a full nights sleep. The clock dial should then be covered, and from now on any other clock in the room that is visible from the bed should either be removed, covered or turned away so that it isn't visible from the bed. This is so that the trainee doesn't adapt to a single specific time to wet, and that the only solid trigger for wetting is the alarm. Every day, choose an alarm at random to set. When the trainee has gone to bed, the alarm will wake them. They will then turn off the alarm and wet, moving as little as possible, then go back to sleep. This will be repeated every night until the end of the training. What this does is establish a new behavior. That behavior is conscious wetting at night. The key point is to get the trainee to sleep, then wet, then sleep. At first the behavior will be difficult. There will be many sleepless nights, and early on there will be anticipation and insomnia. But as time passes and the trainee gets used to the schedule, they will fall into a regular sleep cycle. Later in this phase the adaptation to the nightly disruption may result in automatically return to sleep without wetting. This behavior should be punished appropriately. As long as the alarm is set the trainee should always wake wet in the morning. By the end of this phase, the trainee should be wetting every night consistently without requiring punishment. If this is not the case, repeat the phase until it is so.

Phase 2 - Maintaining Behavior Under Differing Conditions - 1 month duration

The first phase is to establish the night wetting behavior. This second phase is to establish comfort and acceptance of this new behavior. A bedwetter is a person that wets in their sleep, regardless of what they are wearing. At this point, we don't have a bedwetter, but a person that wets a diaper at the sound of an alarm. Consider the different clothing variations that the trainee might experience when sleeping. So far they've been wearing diapers. But maybe they have cloth and disposable diapers. What if they were wearing regular underwear? Or all these variations fully clothed, or completely nude. Once the variations are figured out, set a random schedule, and continue the use of the alarm clock-wetting routine with the added variation of the different conditions. Keep in mind that this phase requires the most cleaning, make sure that you have many extra sets of sheets and the mattress is protected. Now that the new behavior has been established it is still, unfortunately, a specific habit: The trainee has so far been trained to wet a diaper at night. What the trainee needs is to be comfortable wetting and being wet. This phase helps the trainee to learn to be comfortable in a wet bed, or wet clothes and still able to return to a sleeping state. If by the end of the month the trainee is still having trouble returning to a regular sleep cycle, repeat the phase until they have done so.

Phase 3 - Weaning and Reward - 12-week minimum duration

At this point, the trainee has spent at least two months consistently wetting at night. In the mind of the trainee two things have happened, the behavior has become a habit, and the brain has gotten used to urinating during the three-hour alarm period at night. By repetition we are creating the urge to urinate during this period even though the trainee has most likely not yet felt that urge because of the alarm. This phase is the trickiest part of the training. Up until now the trigger for wetting has been the alarm. Now we turn off the alarm. But it can't be done all at once. So, the trainee must be weaned slowly off the alarm until it becomes unnecessary. Start by randomly selecting one night of the week. This will be the night the alarm won't be activated. A random day will be chosen for the next two weeks, and ideally every two weeks the number of days per week that the alarm is inactive will increase by one until after twelve weeks the alarm is no longer necessary. Because this phase can be extremely tricky be prepared to delay progress or even return to phase 2 until the desired behavior is achieved. The child's wetting calendar will come in handy at this point as it will be easy to track the trainee's progress. The behavior that is desired is that on nights that the trainee doesn't experience the alarm, they will still wet. Realistically there are three possible scenarios when the alarm is off: The trainee sleeps through the night, the trainee wakes because of the established habit of waking at this time, or the trainee doesn't wake but still wets. If the trainee should wake, they should wet before returning to sleep. Early in this phase don't worry if the trainee sleeps through the wetting period, however, don't progress with the weaning if the trainee hasn't wet after the first four weeks. When the trainee does wet, either by waking or sleeping, reward the behavior. Show the trainee that this is the desired behavior and that it will be rewarded, and the trainee will have a greater incentive to continue the behavior. In this way also, the mind of the trainee will be conditioned to want to wet. As the wetting behavior continues without the alarm, the trainee will require waking less and less. As it is, with the alarm activated, after so long the trainee ought not even need to stay awake, but might even be falling asleep while wetting after having experienced the situation so many times. So now with the alarm inactive the sleep wetting has a chance to occur naturally. By the seventh to eighth week, the randomized condition training begun in the second phase can end provided the trainee has shown the ability to wet in each of the conditions without the alarm. Once the trainee has been able to wet, awake or asleep, without the alarm at least 50% of the time this phase can end after at least two weeks of only one night where the alarm is activated per week.

Phase 4 - The Bedwetter and Diminishing Returns

At this point, the trainee has established the ability to wet at night without the need for an alarm. As well because the alarm is no longer being used, most of the time the trainee should be wetting without waking. However, this is also taking up a lot rewards. But since the trainee is now a bedwetter, they don't need the rewards. But still we can't just stop, so like the alarm we must ween the trainee. At the start of this phase we change the reward scheme to only reward nights where the trainee has only wet in their sleep. Do that for several weeks. Keep in mind the wetting calendar will be very handy at this point. Once the trainee has gotten used to this new reward scheme reduce the reward period from one night to two nights. After several weeks reduce it again to three nights. Every few weeks keep reducing the rewards until it takes a full week to wet. This will wean the trainee off the rewards, but it will also encourage more wetting since the mind of the trainee is conditioned to be rewarded for wetting. At this point don't end the rewards all together but keep it up for the next month or so in order to continue or encourage the wetting behavior. The rarity of reward will encourage greater regularity of the wetting behavior. When the trainee is wetting 75% of the time or more should the rewards end, and the training period officially ends.

A Word on Punishment and Reward

Notice that when I mention punishment I said "this behavior should be punished appropriately. I am not a proponent of harsh punishments, nor do I pretend to know all the various dynamics that might come into play between *trainee* and *trained*, or even trainee by themselves. Punishment need only be as harsh as necessary to be effective, and the trainer ought to know best what is the most effective punishment. No punishment should result in injury. Rewards can be tricky. As often as a trainee might wet the bed, it will be difficult to reward with stuff, because that could be expensive in the long term. I recommend sensory rewards like pleasure or even orgasm, but that implies a greater control and specific relationship on the part of the trainer. As with punishment the trainer has the best understanding of the trainee and the nature of their relationship. Reward appropriately.

Appendix five: A personal thought

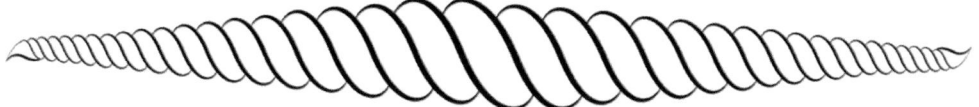

I've been on a journey to become a bedwetter, and I know many others have the same interest. In thinking it through, I see several key elements that describe the road to becoming a bedwetter. This framework can create a profile of where you are on your journey and create a profile of where you want to be. This profile may be useful for describing yourself to others, but more importantly, can force thought about where you really want to be and the barriers to getting there. Hope this helps, feel free to add or modify.

The key elements are the type of wetting, frequency, and ease of wetting.

Types:
Conscious wetting - Peeing the bed or your diapers either before going asleep or when you awaken in the middle of the night.
*Situational incontinence** - Peeing the bed or diapers while asleep, but only occurring when the "stage is set" such as having a protected bed and/or having a diaper on
Involuntary bedwetting - Peeing the bed no matter what, even without a diaper or protected bed. This includes all situations, even when it's inconvenient (during family vacations, visiting relatives etcetera)

Frequency:
1- Rarely, less than once a month
2- Once every couple of weeks
3- Usually every week
4- Several nights a week
5- Rarely a dry night

Ease:

Difficult - Results typically require extraordinary measures such as massive fluid intake, hours without restroom before bed, heavy drinking (not advised)

Moderate - Results typically require moderate measures such as not going to the restroom before bed, reasonable amount of fluids throughout the day, potentially sleep supplements or light drinking

Easy - Results occur with no extraordinary efforts, wetting may occur even if you've gone to the restroom right before bed and without any drinking / supplements

For anyone who is curious, my current state seems to be Situational Incontinence, several nights a week, moderate to somewhat easy. Like many, I want to be at Involuntary, 4-5 frequency and easy. I'm indicating it "seems" such because I may have some involuntary bedwetting. Since I truly wet in my sleep several nights a week, I always diaper up (even on family vacations) This makes it a little trickier to determine if it's involuntary or not. Several months ago, I slept without a diaper and awoke dry which makes me think I may not be involuntary yet (I'm at this contradicting stage where I am happy with wet sheets if it's from over-wetting my diaper while asleep, but don't like wetting my sheets when I'm awake. A barrier of sorts for me is that it is hard to release when I awaken in the middle of the night if I know it's going to wet the sheets. This is probably the final barrier to me becoming an involuntary bedwetter, like all of the previous barriers I'm sure I can overcome it if I decide to). Oddly enough I might actually be involuntary now anyways, I don't actually know!

* Situational incontinence, a term I hadn't heard of until I read through Rosalie Bent's "There's still a baby in my bed!", highly recommended. Even as a DL I got a lot out of her book.

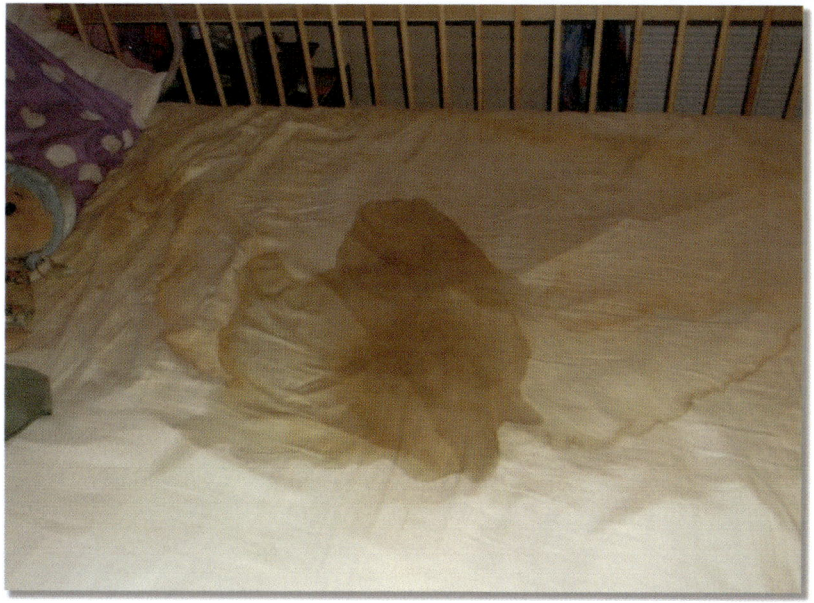

What do I do next?

Go to www.abdiscovery.com.au to see exhibitions of extended bedwetting as well as other bedwetting books and compendiums! There are even bedwetting competitions!

Now that you have read this book you might be interested in more of Forrest Grant's books. Go to https://abdiscovery.com.au/forrest-grant/ to find more of his work. You will also find our complete collection of AB fiction and non-fiction.

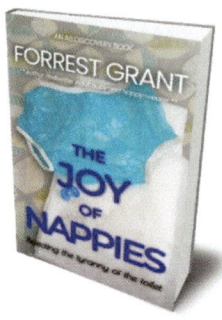
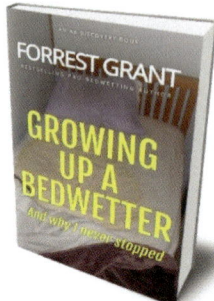
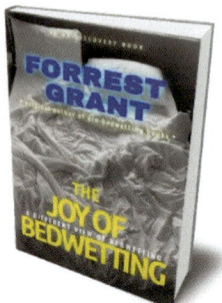
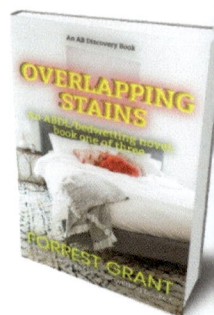

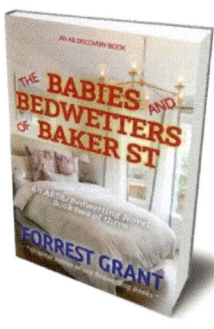
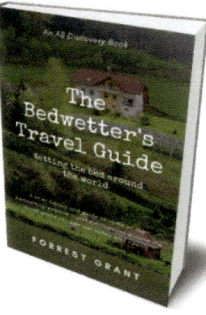
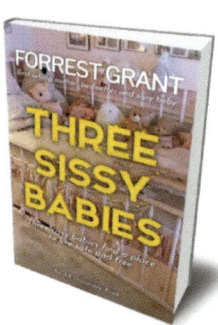

Printed in Great Britain
by Amazon